EBURY PRESS

BACK TO THE ROOTS

Luke Coutinho is a globally renowned holistic lifestyle coach in the field of integrative and lifestyle medicine. His approach towards prevention and healing revolves around four important pillars: balanced nutrition, adequate exercise, quality sleep and emotional detox.

He has also authored a range of books on lifestyle and wellness and has three bestsellers to his credit: *The Great Indian Diet* with Shilpa Shetty, *The Dry Fasting Miracle—From Deprive to Thrive* with His Highness Sheikh Abdulaziz Bin Ali Bin Rashid Al Nuaimi, member of the Ruling Family of Ajman, and *The Magic Weight-Loss Pill* with Anushka Shetty. His most recent digital releases are *The Magic Immunity Pill: Lifestyle* with Shilpa Shetty and *A New Way of Living*.

Tamannaah is a popular model and actor. She has worked in several blockbuster Tamil and Telugu films, and was widely acclaimed for her role in *Baahubali* which broke all records at the box office. She has acted in nearly sixty-five films in three languages.

T0158271

BACK
TO THE
ROOTS

CELEBRATING INDIAN WISDOM AND WELLNESS

LUKE COUTINHO WITH TAMANNAAH

EBURY
PRESS

An imprint of Penguin Random House

EBURY PRESS

USA | Canada | UK | Ireland | Australia
New Zealand | India | South Africa | China

Ebury Press is part of the Penguin Random House group of companies
whose addresses can be found at global.penguinrandomhouse.com

Published by Penguin Random House India Pvt. Ltd
4th Floor, Capital Tower 1, MG Road,
Gurugram 122 002, Haryana, India

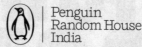

First published in Ebury Press by Penguin Random House India 2021

Copyright © Luke Coutinho and Tamannaah Bhatia 2021

All rights reserved

10 9 8 7 6 5 4 3 2 1

ISBN 9780143455165

Typeset in Adobe Caslon Pro by Digiultrabooks Pvt. Ltd
Printed at Thomson Press India Ltd, New Delhi

www.penguin.co.in

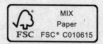

Contents

To Narendra Modi and his Fit India Movement. A visionary leader who has recognized the importance of health and lifestyle and is doing what he can, through us, the people, to improve our health.

I also dedicate this to my family, and my daughter, Tyanna, a constant reminder that life is beautiful.

We dedicate this to every citizen of India, our great nation; be proud of your history and heritage, and the wisdom of our elders.

We dedicate this to every citizen across the globe.

Preface

As much as our world has advanced, we must not ignore the wisdom of our ancestors—those who used nature and simplicity to recover from illness, prevent sickness, and live healthy and happy lives.

Sickness and death can strike anyone at any time. But that is not an excuse to ignore our health, abuse our hearts, minds and physical selves with a poor lifestyle. What does a healthy lifestyle consist of? Natural, healthy food in the right quantity and at the right time; movement and exercise; quality sleep; emotional health and wellness; ample sunlight; happy relationships; happy thoughts, kind words; a spiritual path; yoga, pranayama (breath control); making memories; giving back from our hearts . . . all of this is beyond pills and drugs. But nothing is more powerful than making lifestyle changes, and investing in your incredible body along your life journey.

Across the globe, the most complicated cases of mine have been solved using the simplest of lifestyle changes in conjunction with modern medicine. Are we against allopathy? Absolutely not; it can change and save lives. Is allopathy alone the answer? No. It has to work along with the patient's lifestyle changes. Allopathy treats symptoms; but integrative and lifestyle medicine will address the root cause as well.

Let me give you a simple example. You have a recurring headache. You keep popping pills as a quick fix. Of course, you feel better because that's how pills work. Soon, you start having kidney problems because of all the painkillers. Now you still have a headache *and* a kidney problem. When you initially took the pill to feel better, did you think about the root cause of the headache? Maybe it was constipation? Maybe it was a lack of hydration? Lack of sleep? Too much stress? If you had addressed the root cause, you would have cured the headache, side-stepped the pills and your kidney would have been safe.

Back to the Roots resurrects our tremendous and ancient knowledge, backed by modern science, to show us how inexpensive it is to invest in our lifestyles, and take our health to the next level. This book aims to show us how to prevent diseases, improve the longevity and quality of life. To show us how easy it is to reduce common pains.

We must always support locals as our first preference, but you should be open to international foods if they have a particular benefit for your health condition, and not be rigid. For example, kiwifruit is one of the best scientifically documented foods to help DNA repair. So I do recommend kiwifruit to my patients undergoing chemotherapy and radiation. We must be open to foods that don't grow in our country if they can satisfy health benefits in a scientific manner.

I am so happy to put this book together with Tamannaah. Shimpli, my head nutritionist, and I had the privilege of working with Tamannaah, and helping her on her journey towards a healthy lifestyle. Tamannaah is such a humble, down-to-earth girl, willing to learn, with immense levels of self-discipline and consistency. A pure soul with a beautiful heart.

As we embarked on this journey of simple lifestyle changes and homely nutrition plans, formed from the wisdom handed down over generations (moms, dads, grandparents, great-grandparents), we decided to put it all in a book and share it with you.

Harshala, my amazing nutritionist and head of yoga therapy, helped us organize our thoughts and ideas for this treasured piece of work.

What you read in this book has had a positive impact on the lives of millions across the globe, irrespective of their nationality and age. I hope you will read this with your cup half empty, or completely empty, and share what you learn with everyone in your family and beyond. We grow as we share and we inspire as we teach others. My love to all of you.

—Luke Coutinho

Introduction

Just like every river has a mouth and flows in a natural rhythm, we all have originating points that we need to go back to in order to live ecstatically. Do you prefer eating dal-rice with your hand or a spoon? Would you like to sit cross-legged while having a meal, or straight-backed on a chair? Well, I sit cross-legged! At home, it's quite easy for all of us, but I do not shy away from sitting cross-legged on a chair in a five-star hotel, too. It helps me form an emotional connection with the food. One of the most important details is not just to eat well and live well, but to be comfortable the way you are in any part of the world.

Here's my story.

There is always a reason we begin something new and the only way to do it is to start from scratch. I met Luke at a point when I was tired of running in circles, the constant yo-yo of my weight, the need to stay a certain size (for the unforgiving camera).

I have tried every diet under the sun, but the thing with diets is that they only work as long as you stick to the course. Once you are off, you tend to go back to square one.

I repeat: I have tried many diet plans, and I can tell you from experience, all diets work if you follow them.

What I was looking for was a plan that was personally sustainable and didn't make me feel guilty for indulging, every now and then, in my favourite kind of food.

While settling on a plan, I realized my main issue (and this is a little embarrassing for me to divulge) was constipation. What puzzled me the most was that I was leading quite a disciplined lifestyle to have this gut issue. This got me to comprehend as to how I want my life to be hereafter, whether to live with it or make the right yet sustainable nutritional changes.

There is always a 'why' and a 'how' in every story. The 'why' is exactly what I mentioned, and the 'how' was an interesting discovery. A combined effort of the guidelines I was given (similar to what you are about to read in this book) and serious self-discovery.

Eliminate and Inculcate

We all have patterns. We must continue with the ones that are good, and the ones that aren't need to be loved, accepted, and then of course, ushered out the door, like an amicable break-up. Luke meets you with positivity and energy that definitely provides the first big push you need. His constant ability to focus on the root cause of the problem anchored my journey.

The problems I struggled with had simple household remedies. Detoxification and elimination are everything when it comes to good health, good hair, weight loss, clear skin and anti-ageing. And I was introduced to oil pulling. Now I feel like I haven't brushed my teeth if I don't do oil pulling. It has become a ritual. The challenging part was to train the mind to let go and take a large chill pill so that it could help my body do an efficient job digesting food and keeping my system clean.

I met Luke after a big dietary change. I had turned vegetarian after eating meat all my life. I was prepared for a meal plan, but Luke helped rid me of my addiction to diet soda. Today, all of this is history. Now, I hate the taste of artificial sweeteners, and my cornerstone problem no longer exists. Luke has had a profound influence on how I look at nutrition and, more importantly, the life process around it.

Mantra

I often receive compliments for my skin and body. Friends and fans generally wonder: *What's the big deal? She is blessed with it; actors have it easy, and they have money to access the best treatments; there is barely any hard work.* I do feel blessed, but my health is purely an outcome of natural nourishment, habits, and regimen. The big discipline is to keep moving.

Exercise and yoga have been a huge part of my routine and have helped me achieve balance in life. Even though there are days when I spend long hours shooting, I make sure to cram in a little yoga or a quick circuit to keep the happy hormones flowing. Again, exercise but do not overtrain. You don't have to punish yourself; stay humble, and respect your body. Just because a person your age can do a particular workout doesn't mean you have to follow suit. You have to compete with the reflection in the mirror.

Learn from your shortcomings, improvise; give 100 per cent and leave the results to the universe.

That's what yoga has taught me, and I have been applying this to physical and emotional aspects of my life. Make sure you sleep like a baby; don't compromise on it for anything.

The key is identifying where you are going wrong, brainstorming solutions, and drawing up an action plan with an umbrella of discipline.

Aim

I work in an extremely progressive industry. At times we have long working hours, and there are days that are relatively less hectic. Hence, it is important to understand that the food you eat today will not be the same tomorrow. The amount of energy you expend, the kind of mental strength you use in office, and everything else, is constantly evolving on a day-to-day basis. Then how can one piece of paper, listing food items and a method of eating, work effectively for all of us? It's about time we snap out of all the dreams and illusions regarding diets. Stop being influenced by fancy articles and what the world is doing. Aim for good health. The fact that you've put on weight or you're enduring a particular health issue is because you stopped looking after your body. Maybe you stopped doing what you knew how to do best.

Hope this read makes you one curious cookie as it has made me. Hope it makes you discover that age-old habits were, are, and always will be, the real deal.

This book will help you go back to the roots, soak in the accrued wisdom, and embrace those remedies.

—Tamannaah

A Note to the Readers

They say emotions speak louder than words. To me, India is an emotion!

A rainbow signifies nature's oneness in diversity: an aggregation of diverse yet synchronous colours in the ethereal sky. Discrete colours disperse and turn invisible. By the prismatic effect of the sun and clouds, a magical reflection forms a rainbow signifying harmony and equanimity.

In a similar way, our Indian roots are a beautiful amalgamation of diverse practices.

From an early age, Indians are introduced to habits that are forever engraved in their hearts. They are often told to carry out a certain ritual out of respect for tradition. But most of us remain unaware of the science behind these rituals. There is a logical explanation behind everything; we are simply unaware of it. A lot of the time, even our elders are not aware of the reasons. In the absence of this knowledge, we conveniently call them superstitious or old-fashioned. However, this book offers insights and will help you rediscover all the small habits backed by ancient wisdom that were practised in India.

An honest attempt has been made to present hitherto unexplained facts about forgotten practices, certain commonly followed ones, and the rationale behind them. We hope that readers will find a connection and take pride in what they do and why they do it.

In today's fast-paced world, it is difficult to make time for all these practices. There is a note at the end of every chapter to help you blend these practices into your daily routine.

Let's open our hearts; open our arms to embrace and heal.

It is said that we all emanate from one supreme source and return to that same source: Back to the roots.

—Harshala Chheda
Head of Yoga, Nutritionist and
Lifestyle expert at Luke Coutinho
Nutrition Science, Sports and Clinical Nutrition Specialist
Diabetes Educator
Animal Flow Instructor
Reiki Healer

दीपो भक्षयते ध्वान्तं कज्जलं च प्रसूयते ।
यदन्नं भक्षयेन्नित्यं जायते ताहशी प्रजा ॥

Dipo bhakshayate dhvantam kajjalam cha prasuyate.
Yadannam bhakshayennityam jayate tadrishi praja.

Lamp eats darkness and produces [black] soot!
What food (quality) [one] eats daily, so will [one] produce.

—Chanakya

Let Food Be Thy Medicine

Food serves major nutritional needs, but with growing industrialization, certain traditional practices are being sidelined. The opulence of the working sector, changing lifestyles, and reduced economic provisions for healthcare are a few major reasons why people are turning to wellness. Globally, over the years, there has been increasing interest in traditional medicine. Although India has been successful in promoting its therapies, extensive research and evidence-based knowledge is required. Increased side effects, lack of treatment for chronic diseases, high cost of new drugs, lack of care, microbial resistance and emerging diseases are a few reasons for the growing popularity of complementary and alternative medicines.

India: Birthplace of Traditional Medicine

India is renowned for Ayurveda, Siddha and Unani—traditional medicinal systems. The literal meaning of Ayurveda—science of life, science of longevity—defines positive health as metabolically well-balanced human beings. Alternative medicine or unconventional treatment methods are being used by about 60 per cent of the world's population. These methods are not only used by rural masses as primary healthcare, but are also used in developed countries where modern medicine is the rule of thumb. Plants used as medicine has been an ancient practice and is an important component of the healthcare system in India. An estimated 70 per cent of the Indian rural population depends on the traditional Ayurvedic system of medicine.

Most practitioners of traditional medicine prepare their own formulations best suited for their patients. Approximately 40 per cent of people in Western countries use herbal medicine for treatment of various diseases. With a steady rise of side effects, adverse drug reactions and cost factors of modern medicine, the paradigm is rapidly shifting towards traditional medicine.

Did You Know?

'India is one of the largest producers of medicinal plants. There are currently about 2,50,000 registered medical practitioners of the Ayurvedic system, as compared to about 7,00,000 of contemporary medicine. In India, around 20,000 medicinal plants are recorded; however, traditional practitioners use only 7,000–7,500 plants for curing different diseases. The proportion of use of plants amongst different Indian systems of medication is Ayurveda 2000, Siddha 1300, Unani 1000, Homeopathy 800, Tibetan 500, Modern 200, and Folk 4500. In India, around 25,000 effective plant-based formulations are utilized in traditional and folk medicine. Over 1.5 million practitioners are using the dated medicinal system for healthcare in India. It's estimated that over 7800 manufacturing units are involved in the process of production of natural health products and traditional plant-based formulations in India, which needs over 2000 heaps of medicinal plant material annually.'[i]

[i] Pandey, M.M., Rastogi, S. and Rawat, A.K. (2013). 'Indian Traditional Ayurvedic System of Medicine and Nutritional Supplementation'. Evidence-based Complementary and Alternative Medicine: eCAM, 2013, 376327. https://doi.org/10.1155/2013/376327.

Dinacharya (Daily Routine)

Dinacharya is a concept in Ayurvedic medicine that looks at the cycles of nature, and bases daily activities around them. Ayurveda contends that routines help establish balance, and that understanding daily cycles is useful for promoting a healthy lifestyle.

Lifestyle: A Powerful Drug

We often opt for fad diets when we are filled with insecurity, fear, and desperation to lose weight or cure a disease. If you are one of those who have tried all diets and are still searching for the right one, then by now you know that none of these fad diets work. The only thing that can help you lose weight—and keep from gaining those extra kilograms, prevent the onset of disease, and possibly heal even more serious ones—is a powerful drug called lifestyle.

It is very important to understand that we may not be eating the same kind of food every day, since our body and work keeps changing and so do our goals. In this ever-changing society, it is better to keep the basics right in order to keep going. Working on the basics starts with a core component: Lifestyle.

Intermittent fasting, I believe, is going to replace every single fad diet on this planet because it works beautifully. Fasting is a complete abstinence from food for a varying length of time. Fasting is nature's oldest, most effective, and least expensive, method of treating diseases. It is recognized

1

as the cornerstone of natural healing. The practice of fasting is followed in almost every religion. Muslims, Hindus, Buddhists, and many others have their periods of strict fasting.

The prerequisite, however, is to get weight loss out of your mind. Aim for good health instead. The fact that you put on weight, and are unable to lose those extra kilograms, is because you stopped looking after your health. Embrace this way of life, called Intermittent Fasting. It is not a diet. It respects two cycles in the human body. Every human body goes through an elimination phase and a building phase. It's as simple as that. If you eat in the elimination phase, it's not going to help you with your weight, immunity, or any aspect of your health. However, if you eat well in the building phase, that's when cells are receptive to nutrition. They act as sponges waiting for nutrition, vitamins, energy and trace minerals. That's precisely why it's called the building phase. The elimination phase is when you are detoxifying, cleaning, repairing, rejuvenating and rebuilding. One cannot complicate the two phases.

Structure of Fasting

We can sync intermittent fasting with our biological clock. The circadian rhythm, a natural process that regulates the sleep–wake cycle, is in line with nature. Everything from your hormonal balance to your immune system happens according to your biological clock. Align your fasting time with this natural rhythm and you won't have to change your timings every day!

Let's say you decide to start your intermittent fast at 6 p.m. or 7 p.m. with an intention to eat after twelve hours; then you fast till 6 a.m. or 7 a.m. the next morning. Perhaps go on till 8 a.m. or 9 a.m. until your body allows. During the fasting period you can have water and nothing else. No tea, coffee, green tea, or lemon water. Just plain water and as much as you want. The water should be at room temperature or a bit warmer.

When you break your fast, drink some lemon water before munching on fruits and dates. Your building phase should begin after half an hour. Keeping your health goals in mind, eat what your body needs during your building phase. Do not overeat or starve yourself. Do not try to dive into the building phase. Respect the elimination as well as the building phase, and your life will change in terms of your energy, immunity, hair, skin and weight.

I also vouch for dry fasting. Similar to intermittent, with one added element being you don't even drink water during the fasting phase. You can choose what you want. I prefer dry fasting because I find it easier than intermittent fasting. However, everyone is different, and you should only do what works for you. Begin making this lifestyle change right now and observe how your health changes for the better.

Tammy's Task for You

Start with one day of intermittent fasting. Don't bite off more than you can chew! Try fasting for twelve hours and see how you feel. Extend the hours if your body allows. Don't be hard on yourself!

Benefits of Sitting on the Floor while Eating

Sitting on the floor to eat is an age-old Indian tradition. Sitting cross-legged also resembles *sukhasana* or padmasana, a yoga posture. Padmasana stimulates the lower spine, facilitating relaxation that calms the mind and improves digestion. By keeping our back straight, expanding our spine and rolling our shoulders back, sitting cross-legged combats common aches caused by bad posture. Sit down, and feel relaxed, before you begin to eat.

Standing, and a state of stress, can negatively affect your digestion, absorption and assimilation. Standing redirects blood flow towards your extremities instead of your digestive system. Eat at least one meal sitting on the floor. The back and forth movement of putting a morsel of food in your mouth allows muscles in the abdomen to secrete digestive juices, and helps in quick digestion. Sitting on the floor grounds you, brings a feeling of safety, gently massages your pancreas and stimulates the release of insulin. If sitting on the floor is uncomfortable, eat your meal sitting crossed-legged on a chair, or the usual posture. Sit in the *vajrasana* position for five minutes right after a meal to enable better digestion. According to certain beliefs, when you sit on the floor at the same level as children and animals, it is easier for you to connect with the spiritual side of things.

Tammy's Task for You

- Week 1—Try sitting cross-legged on the floor for two minutes.
- Week 2—Extend it to five minutes and observe your posture.
- Week 3—Sit for five minutes, three times a day.
- Week 4—Try having an evening snack sitting cross-legged.
- Week 5—Try and enjoy one of your major meals in the cross-legged posture.
- Week 6—Enjoy two major meals sitting cross-legged posture without any discomfort.
- Week 7—Enjoy all your meals sitting on the floor.
- Apart from meals, try and sit cross-legged on the floor whenever you can.

Importance of Eating with Your Hands

Eating food with cutlery is a relatively modern practice, but there is a rationale behind eating with your hands.

The actions involved in eating have been derived from mudras (hand positions) that are the basis for yoga, meditation, classical Indian dance, and directly benefits our chakras. According to the Vedas, this practice allows us to connect with food through all our five senses—smell, touch, taste, sound and sight—cleansing them of any negative vibes. The representations are:

- Thumb: Fire
- Index finger: Air
- Middle finger: Heaven
- Ring finger: Earth
- Little finger: Water

When you eat Indian food (roti-sabzi/dal-chawal) with your hands, you feel an unspoken connection with the food that is missing when you're eating with a spoon and fork. It increases mindfulness and makes the entire experience of eating more wholesome, satisfying and pleasurable, thereby benefiting our health, weight and digestion. It helps increase satiety and reduces the chances of overeating.

When you curve your fingers to eat a morsel it forms a yogic mudra. This activates the sensory organs that keep prana in balance. The nerves on the fingertips send signals to the brain that instructs the body to release digestive juices. No wonder food tastes better when eaten with hands!

Unlike when eating with a spoon or fork, your fingers come in contact with your food before you put it in your mouth, you're able to sense if the food is too hot, and you will never burn your mouth when you are eating with your hands. Our body is said to contain a certain kind of bacteria that protects us from other harmful bacteria. When we eat with our hands, this pattern of bacteria is maintained and we are protected from contamination.

Saints and sages believed that eating with your hands made an individual conscious towards food. And consciousness leads to mindfulness, and a better assimilation of nutrients, enhancing digestion, and you leave the table with a calmer state of mind.

With food all over your fingers, you are stuck doing one thing at a time. Happy Mindful Eating!

Tammy asks you to eat one meal with your hands and feel connected!

Benefits of Chewing Food Well

Chewing our food well is a lifestyle change that each of us can start right now because it has a positive impact on digestion—be it indigestion, burping, belching, flatulence, gas, acidity . . . As you all know, digestion begins in the mouth. Saliva has two main enzymes: amylase and lipase. These enzymes aid digestion of carbohydrates and fats in our mouth. The more you chew, the more you spend time mixing your saliva with your food before swallowing, the better you digest the carbohydrates and fats.

The action of chewing and producing saliva also signals the oesophagus and the stomach to start the production of acids and other enzymes which complete the digestion of carbohydrates and fats and simultaneously kick-start protein digestion. Better digestion also equals better absorption and assimilation of food. There are so many people who eat healthy but still look malnourished, suffer from vitamin deficiencies, complain about hair fall, poor skin, arthritic pains, etc. This is because nutrition is more than just what you eat. It's about how the food you eat is absorbed and assimilated, and that in turn depends on how well you chew your food.

Increasing the number of chews per bite increases gut hormone release, promoting satiety by influencing appetite and food intake.

More Chewing = Less Food Intake + Feeling Full = Happy You with Fat Loss.

What happens when we eat hastily? When we gobble our food, we fail to use our teeth to break food down into smaller particles. This sends larger chunks of partially digested food into our stomach. This leads to our stomach producing more acid and enzymes to break food down; work that our mouth should have done. This leads to acidity and indigestion. Furthermore, these undigested pieces of food travel down to our small intestine. They irritate the mucosal linings of the intestine causing gut inflammation, bloating, increased acidity, and they upset the gut microbiome. Ever experienced bloating after wolfing down a heavy meal? That's bad gut bacteria behaving the wrong way, and trapped gases, just because you ate too quickly and did not chew.

Chewing, especially when it's a dessert or fried food, is helpful because you will savour the dish and enable better digestion. The whole idea of being a foodie is to savour what you eat. In order to create a bond between taste and aroma, one has to eat slowly.

How do you form the habit? Dedication. Discipline. Commitment. Practice. Begin with one meal, because if you are used to eating fast, it will be difficult for you to slow down. Involve the entire family. This one simple rule can help everyone respect mealtime. When we eat without intent and gratitude, it doesn't work for our body, but by offering gratitude, prayer and respect, we change the entire energy of the food. Mealtime is a sacred time.

This lifestyle change is simple and free, but it requires dedication, commitment and discipline to be able to bring about the change you desire.

Tammy's Advice for You

- Have a mindful mealtime with no smartphones, television or conversations.
- Sit down, bless your food and express gratitude.

- Take six to ten deep breaths to allow your system to shift from rest to digest mode.
- Start eating—one bite at a time.
- Chew every morsel until it is pasty enough to swallow, and then take the next bite.
- Do not rush.
- Practise, practise, practise.
- Also, try and have one meal with your loved ones, every day!

Realign Your Biological Clock

Going back to the roots is all about aligning yourself with the way your ancestors lived, which is in alignment with nature. The idea is to realign your biological clock by sunset.

Dining early: All you need to do is have your dinner as early as possible, after sunset. If you are used to eating around 9 p.m. or 10 p.m., or even later, try to prepone dinner. This will require you to make a few lifestyle changes but it's going to be worth the effort. Apart from not eating anything later at night, you should also try not to drink a lot of water. This will help reduce the number of visits to the loo at night. Refraining from drinking too much water will prevent avoidable breaks in your sleep cycle, and can help improve your quality of sleep. However, it is also important to listen to your body. It is necessary that you approach this as a lifestyle change and not a fad.

Pre-bedtime regimen: Between dinner and bedtime, try and give up using your cell phones, TV, laptops and other media devices. Exposure to bright light could be a reason why you are unable to sleep at night. You can utilize the time between dinner and going to bed by communicating with your family or partner. You can also read a book or do a few deep breathing exercises. Meditation and prayer can help, as well. You need to know that this change cannot happen within a day or two. You need to train your body to align with your biological clock. Make sure that your bedtime and wake-up time is fixed and followed daily. Discipline your body. It might seem like a struggle for the first few nights, but eventually, your biological clock will reset automatically.

How to plan your meals: People who practise intermittent fasting or dry fasting do not have to worry about breakfast. For others, you need to eat the staple breakfast you grew up eating. It can be idli, dosa, poha, paratha, eggs, etc. Have a satisfying breakfast while keeping a check on the portions.

Lunch should be simple and wholesome. Again, it should be something you grew up eating. It can be simple khichdi, dal-rice with ghee, and a roti, if you want. Your post-lunch snack should be comparatively lighter since you're going to have an early dinner. You can munch on a seasonal fruit sprinkled with soaked nuts and seeds. Avoid caffeine after midnight so you don't hamper sleep quality.

For dinner, you can have khichdi prepared with rice, bajra, jowar, or any other grain of your choice. Khichdi is a wholesome dish that's great for digestion, gut health and much more.

Work towards maintaining the same timings for breakfast, lunch and dinner. This back-to-roots lifestyle plan can help you feel much healthier.

A healthy lifestyle is the magic drug that can help you live a healthy and fit life. The decisions that you make today—in terms of the food you eat, exercise, daily sleep quality and stress management—are all different determinants of your health.

Tammy's Advice for You

- Pamper your skin.
- Talk to your loved ones.

- Read a comic/add humour so that endorphins are high, thus boosting immunity.
- Play a board game that does not involve a lot of brain activity.
- You can also read a book.
- Practise deep breathing exercises and meditation.
- Say prayers or chant.
- Maintain a journal, focusing specifically on positive events and offer gratitude.

Bus Number 11

People are always going on about vitamins. Can I have a vitamin for my hair, my kidney, my liver? Do I need a vitamin for my heart? What about a vitamin to lose weight? We need to understand that vitamins may be required to treat a deficiency, or when you are on a certain medication known to deplete vitamins and minerals in your body. That is why they are called supplements.

I want to discuss Bus Number 11—the two legs that you have—that I often call Vitamin W. It's not a vitamin that you ingest. It's a bus you need to board every day!

Some upsides of walking:

- It requires zero monetary investment.
- You can do it any time, anywhere (depending on the weather).
- It is a super helpful 'vitamin' for every condition—be it cancer, heart or kidney disease—provided you are physically able to walk.

Besides yoga, walking is that one drug that all of us can add to our lifestyle. Whether you are in your thirties or eighties, walking is for everyone. You may not be able to dead lift, bench-press, or try a CrossFit workout, but you can always walk and do yoga.

Nowadays, a lot of people have jobs and lifestyles that are extremely sedentary. Working out every day for an hour doesn't mean that you're active if you find yourself chained to a desk for the remainder of the day. Instead, this simply means that you're sedentary active. Now that's a huge problem because our bodies were never designed to remain inactive for long periods of time. I understand some of you have real problems like corporate jobs that take up a lot of your time, but if there is a will to walk and stay active, there is a way.

Science tells us that even a ten-minute walk is enough to get your circulation going in a positive way for the body. It is enough for you to change your cortisol (stress hormone) levels. It's all about putting ten minutes aside from your busy schedule to make time for your health. If not, you might just spend more time falling ill and visiting doctors. When you walk or exercise, your breathing is automatically regulated which means you start taking in more oxygen. The more oxygen you inhale, the more balanced are your cortisol levels, as well as your progesterone, testosterone, oestrogen, androgens (including thyroxine and insulin). It's all interconnected. If you're lucky and live in a place with access to nature, even better. It brings immediate calmness that will help reduce your anxiety. It's a different thing in the city though, unless you find a nearby park or garden. A ten-minute walk is a great mood changer because when you walk, your body starts producing endorphins. Walking enables you to prevent the onset of diseases and there is a great possibility that your doctor will reduce your medication.

I always work with a number while I walk because like they say, 'You got to measure what you do, and that's what turns into a result'. So, if you have a benchmark of 2000 steps today, make that 3000 steps, and then gradually keep increasing that number every day.

Adjust and set your goals as you proceed. When I am in India, my target is 10,000 steps, but when I am in the US, I aim for 20,000 steps.

You are going to notice a change in every aspect of your health if you add walking to your lifestyle. The human body needs activity; it doesn't need a one-hour workout alone. Don't be dependent on your drivers and domestic workers. They're there to help but don't let that limit your activity.

Take a good look at your life and think of ways you can improve your activity levels. Figure out your own goals that are not based on what people around you are doing. Once you have your goal figured out, aim to achieve it every day. Every time you meet that goal, you're automatically self-motivated, and self-motivation is the missing drug today. So is 'vitamin D'—which is Discipline.

Tammy's Advice for You

Move! Move! And move some more!

The body has a beautiful tendency to adapt. The more you move the more you will be active and charged. And the more you sit, the more you'll end up being a couch potato which is of course not healthy.

While going for meetings, park your vehicle a little away from your destination and walk that distance.

Significance of Lighting a Candle

I remember my grandma lighting the lamp every evening and calling me over for prayers. The candle symbolizes light and keeps the darkness at bay. It signifies holy illumination of true spirit. The candle is used as a prime form to focus and align your thoughts and help you prepare for meditation.

Lighting a candle, or diya, while praying is a common practice to connect with a higher power. It uplifts and expands the energy in any given space.

In many traditions, a diya is lit in the mornings and evenings during puja. The diya is a symbol of oneself. It is made of clay representing our body, has a cotton wick dipped in oil or ghee. The flame of the diya always burns upwards—inspiring us towards higher ideals. The diya's wick symbolizes our ego. Oil or ghee in the lamp equates to our *vasanas*, or negative tendencies. The lamp burns to produce light for all, consuming the oil slowly and finally burning out the wick. When lit by spiritual knowledge (i.e. the flame), the vasanas (oil) are slowly exhausted and the ego (wick), too, finally perishes. We can truly serve society only when we sacrifice ourselves for others like the lamp, by humbling ourselves, by getting rid of our ego. Just like the sun, the greatest lamp, slowly but surely consuming itself for the survival of all earthly creatures. The sun only gives and asks for nothing. That is why it is called the primary source of energy: *devata*, the one who gives.

Also, incense sticks alleviate your mood and calm your mind. They activate your senses and relax the nerves, making you less anxious.

Tammy's Advice for You

Light a small candle, or burn camphor in a lamp, to create a relaxing vibe and lift your spirit.

The Indian Squat

A lot of wisdom lies in Indian culture, yet Indians have been adopting a Western lifestyle for too long. The truth is we are losing the value and importance of our own traditions.

This may surprise you, but I am sure you cannot agree more that Indian toilets are more hygienic than Western ones. No part of your body makes direct contact with the Indian toilet seat thus reducing the risk of urinary tract infections (UTI).

Using Indian toilets is kind of a squat exercise. In yoga, it is called *malasana*, which strengthens your legs and improves bowel movement. The posture stretches the thighs, groin, hips, ankles and torso, toning the abdominal muscles, and improving the function of the colon to help with elimination. This pose also helps regulate one's sexual energy as it increases circulation and blood flow to the pelvis. Using Indian toilets benefits pregnant women as they have to squat, preparing the muscles for a smooth and natural delivery.

Research has shown that stomach-related problems are higher with Western toilet users than Indian ones.

Tammy's Advice for You

Being in an industry where I have to travel to different places, maintaining hygiene is of utmost importance. Also, the food may not always be the kind I eat, so cleansing the bowels is all the more important. I always prefer using an Indian toilet, not just for hygiene, but also because it aids in bowel movement. I call it the Malasana Cleanse!

Tongue Scraping

Tongue scraping, or *jihwa prakshalana*, is a traditional Ayurvedic self-care practice that dates back to ancient times in India.

Overnight, as the body processes everything that was ingested the previous day, toxins begin to form and are visible as a coating on the tongue. This thick coating can either be yellow or brown.

Each section on the tongue corresponds to an organ, making the tongue a roadmap to the body's health. Scraping the tongue thereby gives our internal organs a gentle massage. When you scrape the back of the tongue, the colon is cleansed, stimulating better peristalsis.

Why scrape your tongue?

- Reduces toxin load; preventing reabsorption of toxins that your body worked so hard to expel.
- Reduces obstruction to the respiratory system.
- Reduces bacteria and dead cells from the tongue.
- Enhances sense of taste.
- Promotes overall oral and digestive health.
- Gently stimulates the internal organs.
- Reduces oral malodour or halitosis.

Steps to scrape the tongue:

- Place the tongue scraper at the furthest reachable point on your tongue.
- Gently, pull the scraper forward towards the tip of your tongue.
- Rinse the scraper with warm water after the first flow/scrape.
- Repeat the first three steps, three to four times.
- Rinse your mouth with water and spit out.
- Clean the tongue scraper thoroughly with soap and rinse well. Dry the scraper and place it in a clean place.

Serving Food on Banana Leaves

The most authentic way to enjoy a South Indian meal is to eat off a banana leaf. An array of polyphenols, a natural antioxidant, is concentrated in banana leaves that adds to the aroma of the food and enhances its flavour.

The use of banana leaves dates back to a time before metal became a mainstay. People found it hygienic to use fresh leaves that were disposable instead of wooden utensils. Lotus leaves were also used to serve prasad since the flower is considered sacred and pure in many temples. But they were not big enough for a meal. Banana leaves, on the other hand, were not perforated, easily available, large and thick. They could easily hold curries or chutneys. Moreover, sitting on the floor and eating was recommended as the repeated bending of the spine was known to improve blood circulation.

A number of young people have migrated to a different place for jobs, higher studies, or to begin afresh. For them, cleaning their own plates may become a task and they conveniently opt for disposable plates or eat directly from a silver foil that is easy to discard saves time.

Tammy's Advice for You

I suggest opting for dried banana leaf plates that are abundantly available and eco-friendly, besides adding a dose of antioxidants.

Kamasutra

The Kamasutra is the best-known Indian treatise on sexual love recorded centuries ago. One of the three goals of life is Kama, sensual or sexual pleasure, and Sutra, a thread or line that holds things together. It is a common perception that the Kamasutra is a sex manual, but it is actually a guide to virtuous and gracious living that discusses the nature of love, family life, and other aspects pertaining to pleasure-oriented faculties of human life.

Sex helps you build stronger, deeper and more intimate relationships. Have your dinner early and disconnect with your gadgets one hour before you sleep. This will help your body produce melatonin, the sleep hormone. What do you do next? Make love, of course! Have respectful and safe sex.

Indian Family System

'Feelings of worth can flourish only in an atmosphere where individual differences are appreciated, mistakes are tolerated, communication is open, and rules are flexible—the kind of atmosphere that is found in a nurturing family.'

—Virginia Satir

Vasudhaiva kutumbakam is a Sanskrit phrase that translates to 'the world is one family'.

Indian families are a good example of familial nurturing. It is usually a joint family with three to four generations: uncles, aunts, nieces, nephews and grandparents living together in the same household. They eat the food cooked in the same kitchen, pray together, share a common financial income; the family supports the old; takes care of widows, unmarried adults and the disabled; assists during periods of unemployment; provides security, and a sense of support and togetherness.

Did this bring back a long-lost memory? Contemplate and live this moment. Bring this picture to your mind's eye as you read.

Our first and strongest emotional memories are made within the family. There is an emotional intimacy as one supports others in times of hardship, while celebrating our happiness to double the joy.

Your emotional quotient is incredibly powerful because it puts you in control of your relationships with parents and children, siblings, in-laws and extended family. When you know how you feel, you can't be manipulated by the emotions of others; nor can you blame a family conflict on anyone else. A family that initiates and maintains growth, provides support, security and encouragement to one another, helps fulfil its members' physical, spiritual and emotional needs. There is acceptance, emotional honesty and openness and less room for anxiety or depression, further enriching the Indian family system.

Tammy's Advice for You

You should try and stay in touch with your loved ones—write them a letter or video call them—to strengthen the familial bond, and your emotional intelligence.

Scientific Reason behind Indian Routines and Habits

This section is particularly important so that one can adapt to the practices of the past.

Namaste

Namaste, the traditional Indian greeting! A gesture that displays a deep respect and love for the person we greet. In yoga, this gesture is called the *anjali* mudra. It is a well-known fact that the tips of the fingers are major energy points; when we bring our palms together, the nerves send a stimulus to the brain, leaving the upper body feeling a sense of immediate calmness and well-being. In yoga, each finger represents a certain energy. The little finger, *tamas* or dullness; the ring finger, *rajas* or activity; the middle finger, *sattva* or refinement; the index finger, *jivatma* or the individual soul; and the thumb, *paramatma* or the ultimate soul. This is the yogic definition of namaste.

Significance of Ringing the Bell

I start my worship by ringing the bell, praying that the divine may enter me and all negative forces depart. We all know that traditional Indian worship always starts with the ringing of the bell at a temple.

The bell is a beautifully crafted object made of an amalgam of several metals including zinc, copper, bronze, cadmium, and many other alloys. The quantity of each metal is based on very accurate scientific calculation. When the bell is rung there is an echo that creates an instant harmony between the right and left lobes of the brain; the resonation lasts for about seven seconds touching the seven chakras of the body. The sound of the bell creates an instant calmness, increasing the powers of concentration, and helping you focus on the higher chakra. A well-designed temple bell could also produce the sound Om, the sound of the universe.

Why Do We Visit Religious Places?

Places of worship are built in a way that concentrates maximum positive energy and the scriptures are placed below. The idols and plates of inscriptions are also placed for religious and spiritual needs, and are capable of absorbing and radiating energy. When we visit a temple and walk around, we come within the radius of this magnetic field thereby imbibing a lot of positive energy. That's why a temple visit rejuvenates the body, mind and soul.

Idol Worship

The cognitive power of the mind comes from symbols. For example, when we hold a coin we are aware of the power of money. Certain communities understood that it was difficult for a simple mind to comprehend an abstract truth; hence, idol worship was the answer to unity with a higher reality. An idol helps a devotee focus instantly, enabling the shift to a higher realm. Thus, idol worship served as a tangible symbol for devotees, of various religions, seeking an abstract truth. This enables instant concentration and easy movement to a higher self.

Silk Clothing while Worshipping

Silk has the capacity to create electromagnetic energy. The constant friction of silk on skin creates static. When one wears silk and worships god, there is an instant absorption of this energy that is transmitted to the person, a feeling of instant calmness. Silk also prevents loss of energy thereby increasing concentration.

Why do Married Women Apply Sindoor?

Sindoor is applied not just to indicate a woman's marital status. Sindoor is made from a mixture of turmeric and mercury. Mercury helps decrease blood pressure and enhances sexual drive. Hence, widows were not allowed to apply sindoor. Mercury also helped reduce feelings of stress. That's why sindoor is applied all the way from the forehead right down to the pituitary glands, the seat of all thoughts and emotions.

Why did Indian Women Traditionally Wear Bangles?

It is said that the tinkle of a bangle in a house kept negativity at bay. Ancient Ayurveda stated that the bones of women were weaker than those of men, hence bangles were traditionally made of gold and silver, since these metals help absorb energy which was then transmitted to the body improving its physiological functioning. Also, the pulse was used to diagnose several major ailments in the past (even today, in certain parts of the country); the constant friction between the bangles and the wrist area ensured good blood circulation. The energy released by the skin was absorbed by the metals in the bangles and returned to the body. Bangles were not just ornamental but they also had health benefits.

Significance of Henna

When we talk of Indian marriages, we immediately think of the mehndi ceremony, the drawing of intricate patterns on the hands and feet of the bride. Why do we apply henna apart from the fact that it looks beautiful?

Traditional marriages are long-drawn-out affairs, they create a lot of stress and sometimes fever too; applying henna on the hands and feet alleviates fever and reduces tension, thereby cooling the body. Henna is also an important antiviral and antifungal agent that helps to keep rashes and other ailments at bay.

Toe Rings

Traditionally, Indian women wear toe rings, and not just to indicate their marital status. Toe rings were made of silver and worn on the second toe, next to the big toe. It is a well-known fact that there is a nerve that travels from this toe to the uterus and then to the heart. Thus, wearing toe rings ensured good circulation, thereby strengthening the uterus, and regulating the menstrual cycle that ensured speedy conception. Also, silver is known to be a good conductor of energy; it absorbs energy from the earth and passes it on to the body, thereby rejuvenating the entire system.

Kumkum on the Forehead

Indian women traditionally applied kumkum on the forehead between the eyebrows. Today, it is scientifically proven that this is a major nerve point. The rishis of ancient India understood this to be the seat of the *ajna* chakra, the centre of infinite intuition, automatically activated when you apply kumkum. Kumkum between the eyebrows increases the power of intuition and concentration. It also helped increase blood supply to the facial muscles.

The Indian Tradition of Ear-piercing

Several diseases like hernia can be controlled by piercing the ears. It also helped regulate the menstrual cycle and restrict hysteria. Even the electric current within the body was regulated by wearing earrings. Indian physicians and philosophers believed that by piercing the ears and wearing earrings, there was an improvement in the part of the intellect that comprises thinking faculties and the power of decision-making. It also helped reduce incessant chatter, a process that would drain the body of all its energy making sure that the person was calmer and maintained a certain dignity and decorum. Problems associated with the ear channels could also be curtailed by earrings.

Chanting

Chanting Om helps the mind calm down; thoughts recede, and there is an instant peaceful feeling. Om is considered the primordial sound of the universe—the first sound. This universal sound is a combination of three syllables A (aah), U (ooh) and M (mmm). The lower portion of the body up to the stomach is activated when we pronounce A, the chest area is activated as we reach U, and the face and the brain are activated with the final syllable. The proper pronunciation of Om ensures a good intake of oxygen required for a sound body and mind. Mystics say that Om is like clapping with one hand. Chanting Om ensures peace and quiet that relaxes the body and mind.

Tulsi Plant

In Indian culture, tulsi is accorded the status of a mother. Tulsi is also referred to as holy or sacred basil. The spiritual and medicinal properties of tulsi are renowned. It as an important adaptogenic herb that helps reduce stress.

Tulsi is a remarkable antibiotic as it helps to cure several ailments, including common cold. It doesn't contain other stimulants, thus tulsi helps increase physical endurance. A daily intake of tulsi helps maintain the physiological balance in the body and increases immunity. More importantly, tulsi increases your lifespan. Keeping a tulsi plant at home keeps insects and mosquitoes away, and even snakes, supposedly. In India, every traditional household continues to have a tulsi plant, for both its spiritual and medicinal significance.

Why Are Certain Trees Considered Sacred in India?

Neem, audumbar (cluster fig), and pipal are a few sacred trees in India. These trees are propagated by seeds dropped by birds. Our ancestors knew that they generated oxygen day and night making it vital to maintain the ecological balance. By associating these trees with the divine our ancestors made sure that they were never cut or damaged in any way.

Wisdom behind Eating Sweet after a Meal

Our ancestors stress the fact that every meal should start with spicy food and end with sweets. It is well known that when we eat spicy food the body secretes digestive juices and acids that enhance the digestive process. Sweets contain a lot of carbohydrates which make for sluggish digestion. Also, the intake of sweets enhances the absorption of amino acids like tryptophan. Tryptophan increases the levels of serotonin, a neurotransmitter associated with the feeling of well-being, a familiar emotion at the end of a full meal. This was the rationale behind our ancestors stressing that every meal should start with spicy food and end with sweets.

Why Do We Touch the Feet of Elders as a Greeting?

In Indian culture, it is customary to bend down and touch the feet of elders as a greeting. It is said that by doing this you acquire intellect, knowledge, strength and fame. There is a scientific reason behind this analysis, that the body is a storehouse of energy, both negative and positive. The left side represents negative energy, while the right side represents positive energy. When we bend down and touch the feet of our elders, it indicates that we are surrendering our ego at their feet. This gives rise to *karuna*, or compassion within them. As we touch their feet this energy is passed to us, creating an instant link between the two hearts and minds. The nerves from the brain are spread out through the body and when we touch another person it forms a circuit, thereby transmitting energy from one person to the other. We become the receiver and the other person is the giver of energy.

Do Not Sleep with Your Head to the North

If we sleep with our head facing north we invite evil spirits and ghosts. A myth? Probably. But there was a scientific reason as well. It is well known that the earth has a magnetic field. It is also known that the body has a magnetic field of its own. When we sleep with our heads towards the south then the poles of the earth and the body attract each other. We wake up in the morning with a sense of well-being, of having rested well. Similarly, when we sleep with our heads towards the east, the energy of the sun enters the body via the head and leaves through the feet, leaving you with a cool head and warm feet. When we sleep with our heads towards the west the reverse happens, leaving you with a warm head and cold feet, an unpleasant sensation. When we sleep with our heads towards the north, the iron in our body tends to coagulate in the brain creating disturbances, headaches and unpleasantness. This causes a lot of disorders, including

Alzheimer's, cognitive disorders like Parkinson's and several other neurological problems. This was the reason why our forefathers insisted that we sleep with our heads towards the south or the east.

Shankh

The shankh is small in size but contains amazing healing and vibrational energy! It resembles a mollusc in the sand on a beach. You must have seen a shankh in Hindu households or certain temples. In many households, even today, it is blown while offering prayer. In ancient times, this would be a ritual performed by everyone in the house. Blowing on the shankh creates sattva, pure vibrations! Moreover, blowing a shankh is an art. It has to be blown in one breath thereby improving lung capacity. It emanates the sound of the universe, Om, further adding to the positivity and purity.

It also helps in healing earache. Placing the shankh near your ear enables you to hear the sound of the ocean waves, which can be soothing and is also known to send relaxing signals to the brain.

Throwing Coins in a Well for Good Luck

What was the scientific reason behind this custom? In ancient India, copper coins were prevalent, unlike the stainless steel varieties today. Back in the day, coins were thrown into tanks and ponds because copper made dust particles settle at the bottom, allowing people to collect potable water. Our ancestors introduced this custom to ensure that copper, an essential element, entered our bodies.

Traditional Punishment

Remember when you were punished and made to do sit-ups while crossing your hands and holding your earlobes? This goes back to the days of the *gurukul*, and there was a scientific reason behind this punishment. As you sat down and got up several times, it improved blood circulation, allowing for better concentration and memory power. Crossing your hands across your chest and holding alternate lobes brought about coordination between the right and left sides of the brain. By pressurizing the points on the ear, plenty of brain cells were stimulated thus decreasing learning disabilities in weak students.

Gomutra

Cows are rarely to be seen nowadays due to wide-scale urbanization. However, in the past, nearly every household, regardless of religion, had cows. Cows were being nurtured for their purity and for all that they provide starting from urine, dung, manure, milk and its products. This docile animal was worshipped as *kamadhenu*, the mother of all entities.

The spiritual, medicinal and traditional values of gomutra are very high. Traditionally, it was sprayed in the house to bestow happiness, purity, prosperity, positive health and wealth. Cow urine contains 95 per cent water, 2.5 per cent urea, minerals, twenty-four types of salts, hormones and 2.5 per cent enzymes. It also contains calcium, phosphorus, carbonic acid, potash, nitrogen, ammonia, manganese, iron, sulphur, phosphates, potassium, uric acid, amino acids, cytokine and lactose.

In Vedic texts, cow urine is compared to nectar. It is also mentioned that gomutra helps with certain cardiac and renal diseases, indigestion, stomach ache, diarrhoea, oedema, jaundice, anaemia, haemorrhoids and skin diseases, including vitiligo.

Kitchen Design

Rules in regard to kitchen interiors in the past:

- Kitchens were designed by women to sit and cook at a sigri and not stoves. This way they could avoid getting tired, leading to problems like varicose veins and other spine–muscle–nerve issues due to prolonged standing.

- Food was cooked in earthen pots thereby eliminating mineral deficiency.

- Well water was consumed which was filtered using a muslin cloth to free the water from impurities, and then stored in *matkas* (earthen pots), adding minerals and correcting the pH levels.

- Wood or cow dung cakes were used as means to produce fire for cooking. This helped prevent pollution, and the smoke produced was good for health.

- Cooking used to be done early in the morning and before sunset due to lack of electricity and to avoid insects or pests falling in the food cooked late at night.

- Menstruating women were not allowed to enter the kitchen to give them adequate rest.

- Outside footwear was not allowed inside the kitchen to maintain hygiene.

- It was a mandate that the person cooking should take a bath before entering the kitchen to avoid contamination of food.

- Hair had to be tied to avoid its falling in the food which was considered inauspicious.

- The kitchen was cleaned before and after cooking in order to kill any bacteria and keep ants and rodents at bay.

Self-care

When you see pictures of the ancient times, the lady was always dressed well and looked elegant. She wore kajal and a bindi, had a nice glow on her skin with her hair grown long and thick. Ever wondered how? Since there were no creams or lipsticks or a variety of make-up back in the day.

Let's take a tour on how they maintained their skin and hair health. A large array of various cosmetic ideas for self-beautification existed in ancient India. There was a lot of wisdom involved as these practices were subtly interwoven with the seasons (*ritus*) and the normal rituals of life (dinacharya). Different masks or applications (*lepas*) were used for different seasons. Special oils and ghee were used for facial beautification. Special ingredients were used for hair washes. Many remedies have been formulated for hair growth, prevention of falling hair and premature greying. It appears that modern cosmetic mixtures were conceived by the ancient Indians who utilized naturally available resources.

Here are a few mixtures that were applied unlike today's chemical-based products.

Bindi	Yellow turmeric mixed with lime juice that turns it bright red
White tilak	Sacred white ash
Eye make-up	Kohl
Red colour for eye shadow	Kohl was mixed with turmeric and ginger root

Here are few formulations using natural ingredients to enhance beauty, and remedies for common issues like pimples, cracked lips, etc.

Used for	Formulation
Cracked lips	A paste of powdered bael (wood apple) mixed with milk. 1 tsp bael fruit powder and 1 tsp coconut oil with a few drops of milk.
Depilatory	Pound 1 tsp amla (Indian gooseberry) powder, 1 tsp pippali (long pepper) and soak in neem powder with water.
Depilatory	2 tbsp neem leaves, 1 tbsp fennel seeds, 2 tbsp aloe vera gel, 1½ tbsp green lentil powder, 1 tbsp rice starch, 4 almonds (soaked), 1 tbsp multani mitti (Fuller's earth). Mix well and scrub.
Face pack	1 tbsp red lentils (powdered), 1 tsp raw honey, 1 tbsp homemade ghee.
Pimples	1 tbsp multani mitti mixed with ½ tsp turmeric and water.
Lice and nits	Boil a cup of neem leaves and blend it with water into a paste. Apply this on your hair and scalp. A piece of cloth dipped in the juice of betel leaves and cinnamon. 1 tsp reetha (Indian soapberry) powder with 1 tsp amla powder mixed in water to make a paste.
Dandruff, itching, alopecia, premature greying	2 tbsp juice of bhringaraj (false daisy) in an iron pan with ½ tsp each of triphala, beheda and amla. Cook in coconut/mustard/castor oil.

Deodorant powder	Powdered bark of mango and pomegranate (1 tsp each), mixed with 2 tbsp any flower/sandalwood.
Bad odour	A powder made of tamarind, cardamom and sandalwood.
Skin lightening	Banana skin massage (homemade paste). 1 tsp turmeric mixed with 1 tbsp milk cream and 1 tsp besan (gram flour), 2 tsp rice powder mixed with a little coconut oil. 1 tsp ghee, 2 tbsp ripe banana paste and 1 tsp raw honey, grind fresh orange/pomegranate peels with cold milk. Mix 2 tsp of aloe vera gel, ½ tsp of turmeric, 1 tbsp of honey.
To shrink pores	Mix 2 tsp of cornflour powder and 1 egg white. 1 cup juice of peeled cucumber. To this, add 1 tbsp sandalwood powder and 1 tbsp lemon juice.
De-tanning	Apply raw potato juice. Mix 2 tbsp rice flour with 2 tsp cold milk and make a paste. Tomato juice. Mint leaf juice.
Reduce pigmentation	Mix 2 tbsp pulp of a ripe mango with 2 tsp besan.
Face cleanser	Mix 1 tbsp orange juice with 2 tsp multani mitti to make a smooth paste.
Golden glow to skin	2 tsp of orange peel powder or lemon peel powder with 2 tbsp raw potato juice, 1 tsp of honey and 2 tsp of lemon juice.

Skin toning	Cucumber peel.
Skin smoothness, skin burn	Aloe vera pulp.
Skin irritation and allergies	Powdered khus (vetiver) root with red sandalwood.
Skin smoothening	Red rose petals mixed with milk cream.
Acne	Lavender flower mixed with turmeric and water (oily skin).
Skin itching and rashes	Coconut oil.
Wounds, skin diseases, leprosy	Neem: Bark, seed, fruits and leaves.
Facial	Milky juice of unripe papaya.
Remove blemishes	Pulp of ripe papaya.
Split ends	Sunflower mixed with coconut/castor/mustard oil.
Skin tightening	Sunflower powder mixed with yoghurt and turmeric. Add 2–3 tbsp hibiscus flower powder in a bowl. Add 1–2 tbsp rice flour or besan in the same quantity, 1 tbsp yoghurt, 1 tbsp honey and 1 tbsp aloe vera gel (optional). Mix all these ingredients for a consistency of a face pack.
Skin rejuvenation	2 tbsp sesame seeds paste mixed with 1 tbsp multani mitti and 1 tsp turmeric.
Glowing skin	1–2 tbsp turmeric, 1 tbsp sandalwood powder and 2–3 tbsp almond oil.

Skin infection	Tulsi leaves paste.
Skin rejuvenation	1 tbsp each of turmeric powder, gram flour, rice flour, sandalwood powder. Mix well with rose water and almond oil.
Soft skin	1 tbsp of red lentil powder, almond powder, rice powder; 1 tsp turmeric in a bowl and a few drops of rose water.
Bright skin	1 tbsp of almonds, pistachios, flaxseed, cashews; ½ tsp saffron, 12 tsp orange peel powder; add rose water, blend and make a paste.
Reduce hair breakage Stimulate hair growth	Tulsi leaves boiled with coconut oil.
Ubtan (homemade paste) for dry skin	3 tbsp gram flour, 1 tbsp sandalwood powder, 2 tsp lemon juice, 1 tbsp honey, 1 tbsp malai (milk cream) and a few drops of rose water.
Ubtan for dry skin	2 tbsp sandalwood powder, 1 tbsp lemon peel powder, 1 tbsp besan and rose water.
Stronger hair growth	Mix 1 tsp brahmi (Indian pennywort) extract with 1 tbsp olive oil.
Hair dyeing	1 tbsp walnut leaf powder, 3 tbsp henna powder, 1 tsp coffee and yoghurt. Beetroot juice mixed with coconut oil. 2 tbsp henna powder, 2 tbsp besan powder and 3 tbsp curd.

Faster hair growth	Ginger root oil, onion juice and curry leaves juice. Soaked and pounded methi (fenugreek) seeds.
Dandruff	½ cup yoghurt, 1 tsp shikakai, 1 tsp amla, 1 tsp fenugreek soaked and pounded, khus khus seeds (pounded) in milk and apply to scalp.
Hair smoothening	Add a handful of fresh or dried marigold flowers to three cups of hot water and apply on scalp and hair. Hibiscus powder mixed with oil.
Damaged hair	1 tbsp shikakai, ½ tbsp of neem powder, tulsi powder, rose petal powder, fenugreek powder, along with 1 cup of curd and 1 tbsp of olive oil.
Shampoo	Reetha powder can be mixed with warm water to form a paste which can be used to massage the scalp.
Hair conditioner	2 tbsp sage mixed with water.
Hair cleanser	Shikakai.

Natural beauty care products were the secrets of glowing and healthy skin and hair in the past. Don't you feel you should adapt to various formulations and pamper yourself? Let's go back to the roots and embrace its wisdom.

Nature Heals

One major difference between our current lifestyle and that of our past is an increasing distance from natural settings due to urbanization. Does this really have a difference on our emotional and mental health? The allure of vacations to beautiful national parks, the joy of camping, or even going on walks at a nearby park to clear the mind—speaks volumes about nature's soothing power.

It is found that people who take nature walks have reduced activity in a particular brain region, the subgenual prefrontal cortex. This area of the brain is associated with rumination, or worrying on the same issues over and over, a common problem in depressive and anxiety disorders.

In my experience, I have also found a positive difference in PET scans of my cancer patients.

In a world where our brains are working overtime and we are shadowed by stress, exposure to nature gets us out of our heads, with long-term, positive benefits. In the hyper-urban world to come, designing accessible, safe green spaces may help the mental health of the population, and also preserve our natural landscapes to be enjoyed by our descendants, which will continue to be a national imperative. In the meantime, a prescription for a nice weekend hike could bring some very real brain benefits.

Tammy's Advice for You

This monsoon, I've been going for a lot of runs in the rain. I have experienced a surge in my personal well-being. It feels like rejuvenative spa therapy. I feel lighter and full of energy. People say that rainwater is bad for the hair but my hair has gotten healthier. Every time I've done a workout run in the rain, I've experienced an endorphin rush and I sleep like a baby.

In one of our many conversations, Luke and I discovered our common love for sunbathing and sun-gazing. It's beyond fantastic! Sunbathing and sun-gazing has made me more energetic and alert. It's no surprise that the sun is called our primary source of energy.

Mother Nature's goodness is organic and real, and I strongly urge you to simply spend some time amidst nature. Even five minutes a day can make a huge difference.

Diversity

Diversity of Salt in India

We can't imagine our food tasting as good as it does if it lacked salt. Salt serves many other purposes apart from just making our meals delicious. Since we have become more aware of what we consume these days, and what health benefits we can acquire from everything we eat, the consumption of salt and its benefits confuse a lot of people. Many studies show that its consumption is good for us, while a few others have shown otherwise. So, it's fair to feel a little bewildered.

So, is salt bad for us?

Salt isn't bad for our body. Although, salt that is refined and present in highly-processed food is bad and too much of it can lead to certain problems. The right salts come with a bunch of benefits for our health and cellular metabolism. It depends on how much of a particular salt you have been consuming.

Contrary to what a lot of people believe, white salt—sodium chloride/NaCl—is a bodily requirement. However, you shouldn't be consuming the kind that is too refined or bleached. It must also be noted that saltless diets can actually be quite detrimental to your health, and end up messing with a lot of bodily functions. A saltless diet can lead to thyroid issues, iodine deficiency, and it can also hamper the growth and development of kids.

It's ideal to use a mix of white and rock salts (also known as Himalayan salt), so that our bodies can receive a variety of trace minerals. A good ratio would be 70 per cent pink salt and 30 per cent white salt.

What exactly is the role of salt in our bodies?

Salt plays a vital role in maintaining our overall health as the main provider of sodium and chloride in our diet. It's also needed for the proper functioning of nerves and muscles. Some other bodily uses of salt are:

- Electrolyte balance: Salt is the main contributor of sodium in our body. Potassium, sodium, and calcium are electrolytes required for the normal functioning of our cells and organs.

- Flavouring and seasoning: It goes without saying that our food, no matter how many spices we use or in whichever way we cook it, would taste pretty bland without any salt. From non-vegetarian to vegetarian dishes, irrespective of the cuisine that we are talking about, salt is the most essential ingredient of cooking and seasoning; without which good food would cease to exist.

- Disinfectant: Owing to its anti-bacterial properties, salt has been used since the old days as a disinfectant as well as a preservative. Salt can also kill some bacteria by sucking out the water from them.

- Alkalizes the system: A salt rich in minerals, like pink or black salt, is alkaline in nature, which makes it helpful in reducing acidity and for the regulation of bowel movements.

What are the different types of salt that can be beneficial for the body?

Pink Salt and Rock Salt

One of the healthiest and most recommended salts is pink salt or Himalayan salt. It is hygienic, unrefined, and has a slightly lower sodium content than table salt. Rock salt also contains trace amounts of iron oxide (which gives it its pink colour) and small amounts of magnesium, iron, calcium and potassium. It's great for the body's digestion process, and also helps in cleaning out toxicity. It contains eighty-five trace minerals that are very essential for your immunity.

Adding rock salt to your diet is a great lifestyle change, particularly for those who suffer from high blood pressure. It benefits your muscles, heart, liver, kidney, and brain. A pinch of pink salt in water also acts as a great pre-workout drink. It not only helps with aches and cramps, but also reduces water retention in the body.

However, rock salt doesn't suit everyone. If you have high potassium levels in the body (hyperkalaemia), kidney-related problems, thyroid issues, or an iodine deficiency, then rock salt might not be the perfect solution for you.

Black Salt

Black salt is popular for being more flavoursome and pungent. It's highly recommended in Ayurvedic texts for better immunity and health. The alkaline properties of black salt can help reduce acidity and decrease the damage caused by acid reflux. It can also act as a great laxative and helps regulate bowel movements. Black salt is cooling in nature which is good for the stomach's lining.

Apart from all these qualities of black salt, it also helps reduce bloating by reducing water retention in the body. Like pink salt, black salt also happens to be rich in potassium and can help people with potassium deficiency. It improves digestion and balances the production of acids and bile juices in the stomach. It also helps stimulate the appetite and is anti-flatulent in nature.

How Can You Control Salt Intake?

Some of the ways of controlling your salt intake is by reducing the consumption of refined and processed foods. While salt is an integral part of flavouring, you can also explore other ingredients like spices, herbs, tamarind, kokum, kaffir lime leaves, lemongrass, bay leaf, etc. so as to reduce the dependency on salt. Another very useful trick is to remove salt shakers from your dining table. If it's not within easy reach, its consumption can go down.

It's understandable to have concerns about salt and its intake. Too much of anything can end up being really bad for our body. Salt should be used in adequate amounts only, without depending too much on white or highly-processed salts. And since it does aid a number of bodily functions and processes, it's a good idea to give pink or black salt a try!

For best benefits, one can try a mix of white salt and pink salt (in the absence of any health conditions).

Diversity of Fats/Oils in India

Coconut Oil

Coconut oil is one of the most amazing gifts of nature. Its therapeutic effect on the human body is beyond imagination. Right from weight loss, thyroid, Alzheimer's, Parkinson's to cancer and cardiovascular ailments, coconut oil has the capacity to heal the body of every disease from head to toe.

This power is owing to its unique structure and composition.

Firstly, medium-chain triglycerides (MCTs) are metabolized in a pretty unique way. They are digested by the liver and converted to energy.

Secondly, coconut oil contains lauric acid. Many diseases today are caused by the overgrowth of bad bacteria, fungus, viruses and parasites in the body. To fight that, coconut oil contains lauric and caprylic acid that supports the immune system, encouraging cellular growth and repair, and has antibacterial, antiviral, antifungal and anti-parasitic properties.

Thirdly, coconut oil is known for its heat stability. It can withstand high temperatures and is recommended for Indian cooking without causing heat damage.

Here are some head-to-toe benefits of coconut oil:

- Coconut oil is great to treat hair that is frizzy, dry, tangled, rough and lacklustre. It can also be used to treat lice infestation and dandruff.

- The brain is one of the fattiest organs in the human body, so it's obvious that the brain loves coconut oil. A magic mix of turmeric with black pepper and 1 tbsp cold pressed coconut oil can help prevent brain disorders; this mixture can help improve cognition, memory and retention, and repairs neuron activity in brain cells.

- Thanks to its antibacterial property, coconut oil is a fantastic hack to fight candida. Oil pulling is an ancient Ayurvedic technique that involves swirling 1 tbsp of coconut oil first thing in the morning. A regular habit of oil pulling goes a long way in preserving the health of your pearly whites, fights candida, bad breath, chapped lips, sores, and removes the whitish layer that accumulates on the tongue over time due to toxins, thereby sharpening the taste buds. This is because of the saponification (detergent effect) exerted by the oil that draws toxins towards itself.

- 1–2 tbsp of cold pressed coconut oil a day can actually work like medicine for an underactive thyroid.

- Coconut oil is the good kind of fat, the saturated fat that helps lower LDL and TGL, and increases HDL. Pure coconut oil is also anti-inflammatory and antioxidant in nature. It helps maintain heart health and reduces plaque build-up.

- Coconut oil helps repair gut lining, kills bad bacteria (like candida, H. pylori) thriving in the colon and also banishes constipation, another root cause of many diseases today.

- Due to its antiviral, anti-parasitic and detoxifying effects, coconut oil helps protect the liver.

- A regular hot coconut oil massage left overnight can provide some relief. It is a penetrative oil that can reduce inflammation and improve mobility.

- Coconut oil is a one-stop solution for our feet, one of the most neglected parts of our body. It can help with cracked feet, fungal infection in nails, athlete's foot, callouses, heel spurs, excessive sweating and stinky feet because of bacterial growth.

- Dryness, scaly skin, psoriasis, eczema, urticaria, vitiligo, rashes, mosquito bites, stretch marks, fungal infections, coconut oil covers it all.

- Coconut oil is a natural make-up remover as well as a natural sunscreen. Along with a good diet, applying coconut oil can help keep the skin moisturized.

- Coconut oil improves our metabolism by creating a thermogenic effect.

- Coconut oil helps in healing autoimmune diseases right from its root, like rheumatoid arthritis, thyroiditis, autoimmune induced type 1 diabetes, multiple sclerosis, fibromyalgia and lupus. To a large extent, it also provides great relief from the symptoms of specific autoimmune diseases like allergies, inflammation, flare-ups, joint pains, skin rashes and bloating. Since 80 per cent of our immunity lies in the gut, it makes sense to use coconut oil to detoxify the colon to boost immunity to safeguard against autoimmune disorders.

- Coconut is of great help in dealing with post-chemo side effects like low energy, weak digestion, constipation, dry skin, hair loss and muscle wasting. Since it's an energy-dense food, it can help with a patient's loss of appetite.

Olive Oil

Olive oil, rich in monounsaturated fatty acids (MUFAs), is one of the most common household oils, and its true purpose is to be drizzled over salads, stir-fried items or soups. Because of a low smoke point, which means it burns at a lower temperature than other oils, olive oil should be used for Indian cooking.

Some benefits include:

- Improved blood pressure
- Glycaemic control in diabetics
- Endothelial function, oxidative stress
- Improves lipid profiles—decreasing triglycerides, increasing HDL and lowering LDL—keeping your total cholesterol at a healthy level
- Reduces cellular oxidative stress and DNA damage from reactive oxygen metabolites
- Curbs weight gain because it improves taste factor thereby increases consumption of salads, vegetables and legumes that are high in fibre and low in energy density resulting in greater satiation
- Delays cognitive decline and dementia
- Protects liver by improving the detoxification process

Sunflower Oil

Sunflower oil contains a high amount of linoleic acid, a polyunsaturated fatty acid (PUFA), and vitamin E, an antioxidant. It has a high smoke point and doesn't have a strong flavour, which means it will not overpower a dish. The oil is rich in omega-6 and the body needs a correct ratio of omega-6 and omega-3 fatty acids. Consuming too many omega-6s without balancing with omega-3s, could lead to excess inflammation in the body, so make sure you use this oil in moderation. Sunflower oil can be used for deep frying owing to its high smoking point.

Groundnut or Peanut Oil

It has a high smoke point and is commonly used to fry foods. Nut oils, like peanut oil, can be fun to experiment with in the kitchen. Peanut oil has one of the highest monounsaturated fat content among cooking oils. It's usually flavourful with a nutty taste and smell, and cooks well at high heat.

A study done on 129 participants showed that peanut oil has a high satiety value, and there was a significant reduction in free-feeding intake, an index of dietary compensation.

Sesame Oil

It has been revealed that the oxidative stability of sesame oil is due to the lignans such as sesamole, sesamilinol, pynoresional, sesaminol, etc. Sesame oil is a supplement that has been known to have anti-inflammatory and antioxidant properties, which makes it effective for reducing atherosclerosis and the risk of cardiovascular disease. This oil is often used for its potent flavour; a little goes a long way. It contains both monounsaturated and polyunsaturated fatty acids, though it's not especially high in other nutrients. It has a higher smoke point and can be used for high-heat recipes.

Mustard Oil

Mustard oil is considered a healthy edible oil because it is low in SFA, high in MUFA and PUFA, specially alpha-linolenic acid, and has a good n6:n3 fatty acid ratio. Its consumption can also prevent children from getting asthma, allergic cold and asthmatic eczema; protects against eye and throat irritation, and strengthens our RBC by decreasing cholesterol and improving the RBC membrane structure. The high amount of alpha-linolenic acid present in mustard oil helps to control high cholesterol level and heart disease. Mustard oil does not damage beta cells of the pancreas gland but enhances the activity of beta cells to secrete more insulin to convert glucose into energy. Mustard oil is rich in elaidic acid and vitamin E.

The Goodness of Ghee

Don't you just love it when foods that feel like an indulgence turn out to be super-healthy? What better example than ghee? Ghee can rightly be called an Indian superfood. Ghee isn't only flavoursome; it's full of vitamins too! It comprises fat-soluble vitamins A, E, D and K2. Ghee is a source of helpful fats: butyric acid and conjugated linoleic acid (CLA). Butyric acid is a short-chain fatty acid that fuels intestinal cells and feeds healthy bacteria in the colon.

Ghee is one of the best sources of saturated fats. Saturated fats are the building blocks of brain cells. Including ghee in your daily diet can improve your memory, promote longevity and restore brain balance. Healthy fats in ghee help improve concentration. Ghee is packed with essential amino acids that help mobilize fat and allow fat cells to shrink in size. If your body accumulates fat quickly, then you must consider adding ghee to your weight loss plan.

There are various benefits of ghee consumption. Some of the lesser known ones are:

- It acts as a moisturizer for the skin and oil for the scalp.
- It helps heal cracked lips.
- It works on burns and helps heal wounds faster.
- Ghee actually lowers bad cholesterol and enhances good cholesterol, thus improving heart health.
- Vitamin K2 in ghee reduces calcification in the arteries.
- It improves metabolism, prevents insulin resistance and unnecessary fat deposition.
- It stimulates the secretion of digestive acids and helps in treating ulcers, constipation and other digestive disorders.
- It boosts the immune system, increasing the resistance of the body against various infections.
- It promotes brain tissue development, and strengthens bones, teeth and cartilage.
- It also prevents the occurrence of chronic arthritis.

While purchasing oil look for these markers on the label:

- Virgin cold pressed/wood churned
- Unrefined
- Unfiltered

Diversity of Sweeteners in India

The harmful effects of added sugar are evident. You cut white sugar from your diet, and cells will begin the process of re-nourishment. Controlling your sugar intake will help create the best environment for a healthy immune system and prevent causative risk factors for many diseases, including cancer. Today, there are many substitutes for sugar, but this section emphasizes on traditional sweeteners.

Jaggery

Jaggery is packed with wholesome properties, hence it is recommended by our parents and grandparents. It is often referred to as 'poor man's chocolate' but is loaded with richness.

- Helps dilate blood vessels allowing smooth blood flow, thus regulating blood pressure.
- It is consumed after meals, as it helps stimulate digestion.
- It works as a laxative and helps combat constipation.
- Rich in iron and helps combat anaemia, and hair problems.
- Rich in zinc and selenium, hence it works as a natural liver detoxifier and blood purifier. If you live in a place with heavy air pollution, you can include this wholesome food in your diet.
- Helps in detoxification of lungs.
- To alleviate joint pain, prepare laddoos with sesame seeds, dry ginger, A2 ghee (produced using pure A2 milk) and jaggery.
- Women going through painful PMS can consume 1 tsp jaggery with 1 tsp sesame seeds.
- Power-packed with nutrients like zinc, selenium, iron, magnesium, etc. to boost immune system.
- For cold and cough, one can include dry ginger powder mixed with 1 tsp turmeric and ½ tsp pipramul; mix it with 1 tbsp jaggery and have it like a popsicle.

Honey

Sticky, thick, golden and uber-sweet, made from the goodness of fruit and flower nectar and the hard work of bees, honey is nature's medicine in its truest form, since time immemorial.

It was sumptuous because of its sweetness, and subsequently due to its medicinal properties.

- Honey has an antibacterial effect on several species of bacteria. In diluted form, it works against E. coli, proteus and strep faecalis.

- Topical application of honey helps healing wound infections.

- It is excellent to soothe inflammation of GI tract, namely gastritis, duodenitis, or gastric ulceration and even H. Pylori and peptic ulcers.

- An antifungal action has also been observed for certain common infections like candida.

- Its antifungal and antibacterial activity is helpful against ringworm and athlete's foot.

- Honey is known to inhibit rubella virus and anti-influenza activity.

- Honey is used worldwide for the treatment of various ophthalmological conditions like blepharitis, keratitis, conjunctivitis, corneal injuries, chemical and thermal burns to eyes.

- Antioxidants present in honey include vitamin C, flavonoids, and polyphenolics associated with a reduced risk of cardiovascular diseases.

- Honey helps lower the oxidative stress which may be partly responsible for its neuroprotective activity.

- It can be consumed for low energy, sleep problems and seasonal allergies.

- In comparison to sugar, honey may lower serum triglycerides.

- Raw honey can activate hormones that suppress the appetite.

- Improves allergic rhinitis.

- A daily tablespoon of honey can actually act as an allergy shot (can also be taken by a person who has pollen allergy).
- Honey mixed with saffron works as a natural aphrodisiac.

All the above-mentioned benefits of honey are wasted if it is substandard and processed incorrectly. One must specifically look for terms like raw, unheated and unpasteurized on the honey packaging to be sure of buying the right quality of honey.

Mishri

- Rock or crystal sugar acts as a coolant.
- Contains vitamin B12, an important nutrient.
- It is believed that mishri is good for eyes if consumed along with almonds and fennel (1 cup mishri + 1 cup almonds + ½ cup fennel seeds + ¼th cup black pepper; mix and lightly grind the mixture; consume 1 tbsp daily).
- It also improves brain function when it is clubbed with walnuts (roast 1 tbsp walnuts with 1 tsp A2 ghee, add 2 tsp mishri, add this mixture to a glass of milk to boost brain function).
- Mishri also helps soothe a sore throat when taken along with black pepper and almonds, by releasing excess nasal mucus (1 tbsp almonds + 1 tbsp mishri + ½ tsp black pepper powder + 1–2 drops A2 ghee. Add this to warm water and drink it).
- One can treat impotency by consuming mishri with walnuts and saffron (1 tbsp each of mishri and walnuts with 7–8 strands of saffron, add this to a glass of milk at bedtime).
- If you suffer from nose bleeds during the summers, simply place a crystal of rock sugar near your nostrils

and inhale its smell. Place a huge crystal so that you don't inhale it by mistake; additionally, mix equal quantity of powdered dry lotus petals with mishri, add this to warm A2 milk and consume in the morning. One can also prepare a mixture of mishri in water and put 1–2 drops into the nose to stem the bleeding.

- Topical application of mishri and green cardamom can treat mouth ulcers.

- Take equal quantities of mishri with dry ginger and store it in a container. Take 1 tsp of this mixture, add 1 tsp honey and prepare a small laddoo. Eat one of these every day to treat hoarseness.

- Mishri mixed with neem leaves helps cure stomach ache.

- Mix 1 tsp rock sugar powder in 2 spoons of onion juice. It works as a great cough syrup and is also good for kidney health.

- Mishri is mixed with fennel seeds and consumed as a mouth freshener.

- Mishri mixed with 1 tsp fennel seeds powder and ¼ tsp of green cardamom powder can help treat headaches.

Dates

Dates are proof that nature always wanted you to relish sweet things, but in a healthy manner. Dates, although feared by many in the fitness space, have many benefits for the human body. It's a wholesome food that can be part of most of our diets. Dates are considered as a superfood and are consumed in many cultures and regions.

Let's understand how this amazing dry fruit brings a powerhouse of nutrients and health benefits:

- Rich in calcium, magnesium and potassium, dates help preserve bone density, maintaining bone mineralization and calcium balance, reducing the risks of fractures.

- Magnesium, abundantly found in dates, governs over 300 functions in the human body.

- Dates are rich in iron that helps improve haemoglobin levels and boost red blood cell production hence combating lack of energy, hormonal issues, low immunity, hair fall, pale skin, and risk of abortion during pregnancy.

- Dates are a rich source of vitamin B, thiamine, and is a superfood for a diabetic suffering from neuropathy and tingling sensations in their limbs. Dates improve neurological function, nerve damage, clotting of blood and usage of protein in the human body. Hence, a diabetic can eat them in moderation, 1–2 a day, coupled with nuts/seeds for fat and fibre to lower the overall glycaemic load.

- Dates are often suggested as the first food to eat when one is breaking a fast as it helps in quick replenishment of energy and glycogen that tend to deplete towards the last leg of fasting. When we are about to break our fast, our cells start acting like sponges, ready to receive nutrition and thus dates serve as the best food for our body at the time.

- The antioxidants present in dates reduce bad cholesterol (LDL) and increase good cholesterol (HDL) levels, unclogging the arteries and increasing the chances of preventing heart attacks and strokes.

- It is also beneficial for high blood pressure as it is rich in potassium and magnesium.

- Packed with vitamin C, antioxidants and iron, dates keep the skin moisturized and improves elasticity. It helps maintain a healthy balance of melanin deposits in your skin.

- Potassium present in dates allows a good amount of oxygen to reach the brain thereby enhancing neural activity. Also, regular consumption of dates has shown a slowdown in the progression of Alzheimer's and Parkinson's as it helps in reducing IL-6 levels.

- It contains 23 types of amino acids, some of which are not present in the most popular fruits such as oranges, apples and bananas.

- It contains elemental fluorine that is useful in protecting teeth against decay. Selenium, another element important to immune function, is also found in dates.

- There are various vitamins and minerals present in the fruit that can help improve sperm count and also increase sexual libido.

- Date syrup is an excellent alternative for artificial sweeteners like white sugar. Boil 1 cup dates in 4 cups water for 20–30 minutes, blend it in a grinder and strain it through a muslin cloth.

Diversity of Rice in India

People often say that rice is fattening! If you want to lose weight, give up eating rice, and so on . . .

The thing is that people struggling with weight gain tend to eat a lot of rice, and they eat it at the wrong time, like one hour before bed at night. Your dinner isn't supposed to be the heaviest meal of the day and if you're going to have that plate of rice you're definitely going to have weight problems. You don't eat white rice and get diabetes; you have metabolic syndrome. Your poor lifestyle habit is what brings on diabetes and then overconsumption of white rice will increase sugar levels; it will make you eat more and you will have insulin issues.

White rice when mixed with vegetables or lentils, the way it is served in India, is indeed a great combination. There's fibre and it's a perfect carbohydrate. When you wash off the starch it actually becomes a light carbohydrate. Again, you go back to the traditional Indian wisdom where rice was always unpolished.

Many varieties of rice are grown in India; to name a few: mappilai samba, poongar, ilupai poo samba, rajamudi, kichili samba, thooyamalli, jeeraga samba, gobinda bhog, mullan kazhama, navara, valiya chennelu, raktasali, sali (winter rice), ahu (autumn), boro (summer) and bao (deepwater rice), and many more.

The table below lists some benefits of the five categories of rice.

Type of rice	Benefits
Organic unpolished black rice	Fibre rich, protein packed, full of antioxidants, with essential vitamins and minerals. Highest levels of anthocyanin antioxidants, even more than blueberries. This helps protect the body from heart diseases, and certain types of cancer, and also helps in reducing inflammation. Black rice is also digested at a slower rate due to its fibre content, hence the food stays in the stomach for more time, increasing satiety and delaying hunger, thus being good for diabetics. Rich source of vitamin E and other vitamins. Helps improve haemoglobin due to good iron content.

Organic unpolished red rice	High fibre content. Good source of vitamin B (especially B6), that helps balance the formation of serotonin (happy hormone). Red rice controls blood sugar levels and helps in the production of DNA. Ideal for diabetics because of its low glycaemic index and low carbohydrate content. The minerals in red rice helps accelerate wound healing. Good source of iron, manganese and zinc. The anthocyanin present in this rice helps reduce and control cancer cells. The anthocyanins also delay skin ageing.
Organic unpolished basmati rice	Due to its glycaemic index, this rice can be consumed by diabetics. Releases sustained energy on consumption and has a unique aroma.
Organic unpolished jeera samba rice	Aromatic rice, resembles cumin seeds. Rich in fibre and vitamins. Regular consumption increases haemoglobin levels and immunity.
Organic unpolished brown rice	Rich in fibre and vitamins. Known to increase haemoglobin levels and improve immunity. Effective for reducing joint pains. It increases good cholesterol and lowers blood pressure and bad cholesterol.

Parboiled rice	Retains nutrients as it is cooked with the husk.
	Parboiling the rice turns the starch into a gel which on cooling retrogrades and creates resistant starch (this starch is not broken down and absorbed in your small intestine). On reaching the large intestine, it is fermented by beneficial bacteria turning it into a prebiotic.
	Due to resistant starch, it may not raise your blood sugar so diabetics can put this on their shopping list.
	Rich in antioxidants to protect against cellular damage.

Did You Know?

Unpolished rice retains protein, fat, dietary fibre, oryzanol, polyphenols, vitamin E, total antioxidant activity and free radical scavenging abilities. Hence these properties do not allow for an instant absorption of carbohydrates that cause a spike in blood sugar levels.

The Truth about Certain Ingredients

Is Milk Good?

There was a time when we all drank milk (including our ancestors) without any health problems. So, what has changed about milk that makes it important to reconsider this beverage? It's the quality. There has been a deterioration in the quality of milk and the health of animals that produce it due to the greed and corruption of most food lobbies. Thus, it is very important to create awareness about dairy and dairy products. With awareness comes the power of making a choice and deciding whether dairy is the right fit for you or not.

What Feeds the Cow that Feeds Us?

To meet supply and demand, cows are fed corn and soy, injected with vaccines and antibiotics so that they are disease-free. They are also injected with oestrogen, bovine growth hormone, to produce milk. When we consume milk from such cows, we see a rise in girls reaching early puberty, hormonal issues (PCOS, ER-positive cancers), obesity, antibiotic resistance and diabetes. There have been hormonal fluctuations in boys too resulting in low testosterone levels, stunted growth resulting in mental confusion, early depression, and low self-esteem. Cows are also milked using unethical practices that leads to the contamination of milk with blood and pus cells.

After reading such facts, you may find yourself wondering: How could I ever give up drinking milk?

You are addicted to milk because the milk you have been drinking has a morphine-like effect. When the body tries to breakdown casein (in A1 milk), a chemical component called BCM-7 is released, which is the reason for morphine-like effects on the central nervous system. BCM-7 causes addiction to milk. That's why children prefer consuming milk.

So how do you choose which milk is of the best quality? The answer is A2 milk.

What Is A2 milk?

A2 milk is the milk produced by desi cows that have only A2 beta-casein protein. There are two kinds of proteins in cow milk—A1 and A2—which differ by a single amino acid. Yet, this one difference can change the way the milk is digested in the human body. The structure of A2 protein is more comparable to human breast milk, as well as milk from goats, sheep and buffalo. A2 is the purest form of milk produced by cows that are nurtured in the right manner. Cows are given fresh fodder, clean water, and are kept in a happy environment. As a result, the milk is purer and highly nutritious.

So, when you drink A2 milk there is no gastrointestinal discomfort and your hormones are harmonized because cows aren't given any growth hormones or antibiotics to increase the output of milk.

Khapli Wheat

In India, wheat and rice are major staples. Unfortunately, most grains have got a bad reputation today because they are thought to be fattening. However, there are other factors at play here. The main culprits being the large portions of rice consumed, second is that it is consumed at the wrong time coupled with a sedentary lifestyle, chronic stress, lack of sleep and unhealthy habits, in general. Just the cereals in our diet cannot be blamed.

Of late, people are not too sure about consuming wheat. They feel bloated, flatulent and acidic. The term gluten intolerance has become quite common. This may have become common because of the change in the way wheat is processed. Earlier, wheat was harvested, shade dried, washed down and sun-dried. It was then taken to processing mills where the wheat was ground into wheat flour and then sold to ration shops and grocery stores.

Nowadays, harvested wheat is not cleaned properly. If you soak wheat in water, you will see dirt floating on the surface. Wheat is also not properly shade dried and sun-dried, the two processes that break gluten.

However, we can replace regular wheat with long wheat grain. Long wheat grain, or emmer, is locally known as khapli wheat. However, khapli wheat is not popular because it doesn't give the regular light-coloured roti or chapatti, the staple food for thousands of Indians. It is dark brownish in colour.

Why should you consume khapli wheat?

- There is scientific evidence that khapli wheat is great for diabetics as it has the ability to lower blood sugar levels.

- Emmer wheat has complex carbs that can boost your immunity. It is a great grain for children, adults and senior citizens.

- The gluten molecule is weak in khapli wheat and is thus suitable for people with gluten issues.

- Khapli wheat has the ability to lower bad cholesterol and this is good for heart patients.

- Khapli wheat has twice the fibre and twice the protein of regular store-bought wheat. It will fill you faster and will reduce hunger pangs, thus aiding weight loss.

- Emmer wheat is rich in niacin of vitamin B3, which is great for your heart and cholesterol levels. Emmer is also a rich source of magnesium and iron.

- Pregnant women and those who have recently given birth can also benefit by including emmer wheat in their diet, because of its rich nutrient profile.

- People with celiac disease may find it difficult to consume khapli wheat. If you are gluten intolerant, make a small roti with khapli wheat and see if it suits you.

Tea

To drink or not to drink tea?

Every day I wake up to my mailbox full of questions revolving around Indian chai and whether one should be drinking it or not. Indian chai has recently become a rage in the West and people from New York to California are raving about its health benefits. This spicy aromatic brew has its roots in India that can be traced as far back as the Ayurvedic medical texts.

So, is there anything wrong with the traditional cup of Indian chai? No. It is the preparation that is going wrong. The original Indian chai was prepared in two ways.

In the first one, the antioxidant-rich black tea is the base. Black tea in moderation is extremely potent in reducing LDL cholesterol, neutralizing free radicals and fighting inflammation. One can add freshly mashed ginger that's known for its anti-inflammatory properties and is a digestive soother; cardamom, a common ingredient in every Tibetan medicine as a digestion aid, improves blood circulation and purifies blood; fennel, also a digestive soother; clove, a powerful spice when it comes to the stomach's gut lining, highly anti-microbial, a natural painkiller; and lastly, black pepper that boosts metabolism, enhances absorption of other spices and has an amazing connection with the way the body stores fat. All of these spices are boiled in black tea that people have sipped for generations.

Then there is a second way of preparing tea by adding a splash of milk and a bit of sugar to the black brew. Some people in rural areas even use jaggery instead of sugar.

Either of these tea preparations are not the reason for being unable to lose weight or healing from sickness. Anything in excess is bad. People have four or five cups of tea a day because they're addicted to their sweet version of this beverage. Overconsumption of sugar and milk is what destroys health. In some cases, milk does suit us. Giving up on your morning cup of tea is not going to make a difference. Going from four or five cups a day to two cups a day, reducing the amount of sugar that goes into it, or switching to jaggery, will certainly help. Take it up a notch and brew that black tea with all the above-mentioned spices and you will end up enhancing your health.

Many have that emotional connection with their tea. It's soothing for them, brings peace, happiness and helps them unwind. If that's the reason behind your morning or evening cuppa, then there is nothing wrong with it and you should do that every single day. Emotional health is important and anything that keeps you happy in the right way should not be discontinued.

Rather than blaming that one cup of tea, let us look at larger aspects of our physical goal and see what really needs correction in our lifestyle.

- Being sedentary or sedentary active
- Overtraining
- Overconsumption of sugar
- Fried snacks and biscuits with your tea is also overconsumption. Don't blame the cup of tea
- Poor sleep quality
- Stress levels

If you're stressed and think that one cup of tea is going to help you unwind, please go ahead. Stable emotional health is the order of the day. We need to feel a little happier, a little more peaceful and relaxed. Other than that, if you constantly find yourself stressed, breathe more. Do a little meditation. All of this is going to take care of your health and aid weight loss.

Having said all of this, there are two things we should be mindful of when it comes to tea habits.

1. Don't wake up to a cup of tea.

Have lemon water and a piece of fruit before drinking tea to alkalize the body since tea is acidic in nature. Also, as a rule of thumb, every cup of tea should be followed by a glass of water.

2. Avoid tea immediately after meals.

The tannins in tea block the absorption of iron from food. It's best to keep a gap of at least forty-five minutes to an hour between meals and a cup of tea.

A lifestyle change that you can bring about from today is cutting down the quantity of tea consumed in a day.

You may want to add a bit of sugar (a bit, not a tablespoon), or even better, try it with jaggery. You will not lose anything, except weight!

Water: The Most Neglected Nutrient

We all know that more than 70 per cent of our body consists of water and it participates in the process of digestion. Every day our body produces about 3 litres of intestinal juice, 2.5 litres of digestive juice, 1.5 litres of saliva, 0.7 litres of pancreatic juice, and 0.5 litres of bile. Obviously, this water remains in the system, but in order to keep the body clean, it should be replaced. Also, our body loses around 2.5 to 3 litres of water daily through the kidneys, sweating, perspiration and faeces; our body eliminates toxins and waste through these fluids. If the amount of lost water is not restored, the process of elimination and cleaning will be hampered, increasing toxin accumulation in the body. Water is vital for the absorption of nutrition and to maintain life; without it, cells cannot survive.

Did you know?

90 per cent of human diseases are caused by improper drinking of water!

What happens when there is lack of water in the system:

- Affects digestion and elimination
- Contaminates blood with toxins
- Poses a threat to the body
- Causes constipation, a common digestive problem

If toxins are not eliminated via the intestines and kidneys, they are then channelized and the body tries to get rid of them through the lungs, which causes shallow breathing and irregular heartbeat.

When toxins in the blood get to the brain, a person might develop migraine or headaches. The lack of water will result in dry and scaly skin, split hair ends and brittle nails. The list goes on . . .

It is vital to understand proper hydration. Water is like the elixir of beauty and youth. It removes toxins from the body and helps prevent health problems. Not only is the amount of water important, the way it is consumed also matters. Therefore, let us understand the golden rules of drinking water.

Sit to Drink Water

It is a good idea to always sit and drink water. Balance of fluids in the body is affected when you stand and drink water. Also, the water moves down to the colon quickly, thereby adversely affecting the absorption of nutrients. This can lead to a host of health issues such as arthritis, kidney damage, etc. By sitting and drinking, your muscles and nervous system are much more relaxed helping to assimilate food and other fluids easily.

When you sip your water, your water mixes with your saliva. Now your saliva is highly alkaline in nature and your stomach is acidic in nature for all the right reasons. Your stomach requires a certain amount of acid to digest food, but the problem is when too much acid is produced to digest excessive food or low quality food. We need saliva to travel into the stomach so that the alkaline effect of saliva can stabilize the excess acid in the stomach. One way of getting saliva from your mouth to your stomach is through the way that you drink water. When you sit and you sip your water slowly and carry saliva from your mouth into your stomach, it stabilizes the acid.

Pre and Post Meal Water Drinking

Drink a glass of water (lukewarm or room temperature) 15 to 30 minutes before your meal, and 15 to 30 minutes after your meal. Now if you must drink water while you're eating your meals, make sure it's just a sip or two. You don't have to drink too much water during a meal because there should be enough space in your stomach for digestive activity. Also, too much water will dilute your digestive acids which in turn will affect digestion.

Drink Water as Soon as You're Thirsty

The human body has a defence mechanism and a warning mechanism. It tells us when we're hungry. If we really listen to our body it also tells us when we're thirsty. Now if you are in an air-conditioned environment you need to be a little careful because sometimes you may not get that signal because of the air temperature, and this could lead to dehydration. There are two other indicators; if your lips tend to get dry quickly it could mean that your water levels are low. The second indicator is the colour of your urine. When your urine is a pale white, crystal white or pale straw yellow, it means you have sufficient water in your body. But do note that certain medication and certain vitamins, like vitamin C, can make your urine extremely dark, so take note of these indicators and listen to your body. Drink the right amount of water, accordingly.

Never Chug

When you chug water, most of it just passes out of your system. In order to assist good cellular metabolism and good cellular energy and activity, water needs to be sipped slowly to allow for cellular absorption. Chugging water only makes you thirstier through the day. When you sip water slowly you'll find that you don't need too much water. It's really dependent on your lifestyle the way you sip your water and the kind of food that you eat. Hydration also occurs when you have a diet that's rich in fruits and vegetables that are high in water content. At the same time, when you drink too much tea and coffee these are diuretics in the body. It flushes out excess water and vitamins from your body. So, for every glass of coffee, you need to have two glasses of water to replenish the water that's flushed out. 1–2 glasses of water before having a bath can also help you lower your blood pressure.

Drinking water in the morning cleanses your intestines and flushes toxins out of the body. Add a dash of lemon to maintain the body's alkaline levels. A healthy human body is warm and cold water disrupts thermoregulation.

Just like there's an art of eating well, there is also an art of drinking water well. Today most of us, including myself, are used to chugging water directly from the bottle. But let's try to sip, if we can, slowly. If we don't have the opportunity to sit at that point, stand up but sip your water slowly. Once the water mixes with your saliva and enters your stomach, you'll begin to notice a marked change with regard to bloating, flatulence and indigestion.

Treasures of Wisdom

Tammy's Mantra for You

Sometimes you sit down somewhere, maybe in a coffee shop, at the office, or in front of your TV, and out of nowhere, a thought pops up:

Why am I not farther in life than now?

Maybe you thought you'd have kids by now. A business that would make a lot of money. Or that you would be a well-respected person that makes a difference in the world. Maybe you thought you'd own a house by now. And that you had everything figured out.

But none of that has happened.

In those moments, it's easy to panic—especially if you look around you. It's easy to look at others and compare your own path to theirs. Why are we so obsessed with timing?

This guy was a millionaire by 30 . . . She had her first bestseller by 26 . . . He became CEO at 40 . . .

Who cares? They are not you. But it stings, right? Why not me is a question that rears its ugly head.

Well, everyone has their own path.

I know, that sounds quite clichéd. But you know what another cliché is? Being an unhappy person. Because that's what happens when you try to control your future. Every time you feel that your life is not the way it should be, you're trying to play the higher power.

Give yourself a break and understand one thing: Your work matters.

Most of our unhappiness stems from believing that no one cares. It's easy to feel irrelevant in a crowded world. You wake up, go to work, get back, and watch a web series until you fall asleep. You're just going through the motions.

You forget what your actual job is: to make yourself useful. What's the alternative? Give up? Drink a glass of alcohol and say that the world is messed up? Life's not a road without speed breakers. Maybe you want to do big things. That's great. But you're not some kind of puppet master who can control life. It is important to practise ahimsa towards ourselves and not be so hard on ourselves.

You've got to believe that your work matters. Why? Because it does. It's about your mindset. You need to move and act in a way that makes each breath count.

Sometimes it takes a while to get to where we want to be. But that doesn't mean the journey is useless. And because we're all so obsessed with outcomes, we think that life is measured in milestones. This brings us to another virtue called karma yoga, which simply means do your work by giving it your all and surrender the fruits to a higher power (*ishwar pranidhan*). It's the discipline of selfless action as a way to perfection.

Let's be productive and create an environment of harmony and joy. Productivity is about trying to find a way to enjoy your work and life. You need to act that way. And you need to stop listening to people who are at a different stage in their lives.

So what if this person drives a Porsche? So what if that person bought a new house? Don't make yourself miserable by going faster in life. Put your head down and keep on working. And be a constant self-critic. Try and mould your words by being kind. Let your self-criticism meet kindness. If your inner critic says, 'You're lazy and worthless,' respond with a reminder: 'I'm doing my best' or 'We all make mistakes'.

Stop beating yourself up because you're not where you want to be. Look, your work matters. *You* matter. Trust yourself. Because life doesn't have to make sense. It just has to matter. And if you act like your life matters, it does. Let us go back to simplicity. Let's not march so hard as everyone trips and falls. Learn to forgive and let go. I want you to practice self-compassion. The core to self-compassion is to avoid getting caught up in our mistakes and obsessing over them until we degrade ourselves. Keep moving on to the next productive action from a place of acceptance and clarity.

Heal the Yogic Way

Yoga has become increasingly popular; millions of people in Western societies, as well as in India, have taken up yoga classes. One thing I've noticed across the globe is that yoga classes only offer asana practices in their schedule. One of the reasons could be because most yoga practitioners and instructors are not aware of the real meaning of yoga. Our ancestors have defined yoga as the union of our mind, body and soul; asana is just one limb of yoga. There's so much more to yoga than asanas.

Yoga is a holistic way to align the body, mind and soul in harmony. There are two forms of the human body—the external body (physical personality) and the internal body (inner self). Maharishi Patanjali—widely considered to be the author of *Yoga Sutras*, an ancient Sanskrit text—has defined the eight components/limbs of yoga.

The eight limbs (ashtanga) of yoga are yama (abstinences), niyama (observances), asana (yoga postures), pranayama (breath control), pratyahara (withdrawal of the senses), dharana (concentration), dhyana (meditation) and samadhi (absorption). Yama, niyama, asana and pranayama have a greater effect on the physical personality or external shape of the individual. These four together are called *bahiranga* yoga (external yoga). On the other hand, pratyahara, dharana, dhyana and samadhi have a greater effect on the internal personality of the individual. Together, they're called *antaranga* yoga (interior yoga).

How can you change your vibe?

Ever wondered why yoga makes you feel good? Because it trains us to maintain and be in sync with our breathing. When we step back into our lives after a yoga class, we are better prepared to encounter stressful situations. You are out of sync if you shift your focus from your breathing towards the stressful situation. Many news channels these days have people angrily debating on a particular topic, which is nothing but noise. Now the more you hear that, the more it moves you out of your normal sync and rhythm. Thus, rather than tuning into the rhythm of an angry debate, we should tune into something that gives us peace and joy. This makes our entire being all about rhythm.

Here is a table enlisting a few yogic practices beneficial for common health conditions.

Health Benefit/ Concern	Yoga Practice
Flatulence/Bloating	Pavanmuktasana (wind-relieving pose)
Digestion	Mandukasana (frog pose)
Constipation	Malasana (various squatting asanas)
Acidity/Summer pranayama	Sheetali
Eyes	Sun-gazing, trataka, moon gazing, candle gazing
Hair	Adho Mukha Svanasana (downward-facing dog pose)

Insomnia	Savasana, left nostril breathing; bhramari pranayama (bumblebee breath), unwind
Concentration	Eka Padasana, Sthitprathanasana (prayer pose), Garudasana (eagle pose)
Abdominal organs: pancreas, liver, etc.	Vakrasana (twisted pose), Ardha Matsyendrasana (seated twist pose)
Improve lung capacity	Trikonasana (extended triangle pose), Konasana I & II (sideward stretching pose)
Healthy spine	Chakrasana (backbend), Setu Bandhasana (shoulder supported bridge)
Lower back pain	Shalabhasana (locust pose), Bhujangasana (cobra pose)
Sitting for long hours	Dvikonasana (double triangle)
Stamina	Virabhadrasana (warrior II pose)
Prevent painful menses	Chakki Chalanasana (mill churning pose)
Immunity	Bhastrika Pranayama (bellow breath), Anuvittasana (standing backbend), Ananada Balasana (happy baby pose)
Anaemia	Paschimottanasana (seated forward bend), Anulom Vilom (controlled breathing), Ujjayi Pranayama (the ocean breath)
Varicose veins	Viparita Karni (legs up the wall pose)

| Winter pranayama | Kapalbhati (breath of fire) |
| Positive body and mind | Surya namaskar (sun salutation) |

Chakra	Asana/Pranayama to balance chakra
Muladhara	Bhadrasana (bound angle pose)
Svadhishtana	Utkata Konasana (goddess squat), Matsyasana (fish pose)
Manipura	Navasana (boat pose)
Anahata	Gowmukhasana (cow face pose)
Vishuddha	Matsyasana (fish pose)
Ajna	Balasana (child's pose)
Sahashara	Sasangasana (rabbit pose)

Note: Kindly practise under supervision.

Your Biggest Enemy

We may lose our cool quite often and may have different reactions to anger. But have you ever thought about the science behind getting angry?

There is a small region in your brain called the amygdala that processes information related to your emotions, and which triggers specific reactions in your body.

In this context, when you get angry, your brain orders the release of neurotransmitters called catecholamines (epinephrine and norepinephrine), also known as adrenaline and noradrenaline. Upon release, these molecules provide your system with energy and strength for several minutes, you feel pumped up and your senses are on high alert. They also lead to an increase in blood pressure, an accelerated heart rate, and faster breathing. Your heart muscles contract and your blood vessels constrict and this energy overload causes one to yell or even turn physically aggressive.

How do we exercise control?

The answer lies in the brain, too. The prefrontal cortex. It is the region in your brain that enables you to control your emotions. In short, the amygdala relates to anger and the prefrontal cortex manages emotions.

To be able to keep your cool is easier said than done. It is important to realize that anger is not healthy.

Since epinephrine and norepinephrine constrict your blood vessels and make your heart pump harder, people who are prone to angry outbursts live with the risk of developing chronic high blood pressure and heart rhythm disorders.

Moreover, anger results in a build-up of glucose and fatty acids in your blood. The increased levels of fatty acids can lead to plaques in your arteries. The walls of the arteries thicken and there is a narrowing of vessels because of this accumulation of fats. This can result in a complete blockage of the arteries.

Few tips to manage your anger:

- Start counting backwards from 200.
- Repeat this mantra: relax–calm down–everything will be okay.
- Neck rolls and shoulder rolls are helpful non-strenuous yoga-like movements that can help you control your body and harness your emotions.
- Let music divert you from any negative feelings.
- It's completely all right to say how you feel, as long as you go about it in the right way. Ask a trusted friend to help you be accountable for a calm response. Outbursts get you nowhere, but mature dialogue can help reduce

stress and ease your anger. It may also prevent future problems.

- Diffuse your anger by looking for ways to laugh, whether that's playing with your kids, or watching stand-up.
- Channelize your energy and go for a walk.
- Breathe slowly; remember that the catecholamines make us do the opposite.
- Yoga, meditation and praying might help you relax more often.
- A study shows the positive influence of writing down the reasons for your anger. Maybe you should even start a diary.
- Playing a sport helps you get rid of negative energy.
- Sleep well and for a healthy duration.

Tammy's Task for You

I channel my emotions by journaling. It is a great way to gain perspective while dealing with negative emotions.

Power of Music and Rhythm

The rhythm, beats and frequency of music is a drug that we often use with our patients to improve immunity, reduce stress, fear and anxiety. It also helps improve the quality of their sleep. It is a safe but powerful drug without any side effects.

All of us listen to the different kinds of music we like: classical, trance, hip-hop, rap and other genres, depending on our state of emotions. Have you ever wondered why we have different tastes in music? A song that makes you feel happy can annoy someone or a song that makes you sad can make others reflective.

Do you remember anyone telling you, 'I like your vibe!' or 'I think our frequencies match!' No, these people aren't on drugs or saying anything airy-fairy. It is for real. It is a fundamental part of our human body. We have trillions of cells vibrating at a particular frequency, which can either be wrong or right.

When you are sick, the frequency at which your cells vibrate is different from when you are healthy.

We Are All about Rhythm

Consider our heartbeat. Our heart beats to a rhythm and has a certain frequency, which is sixty beats per minute. Now, when the body experiences stress, the beat and rhythm speed up and could lead to heart disease or onset of a stroke. On the other hand, when our body is relaxed, our rhythm is normal. In fact, cardiovascular diseases are classified into zones based on the abnormalities in their beats: high-risk, medium-risk and low-risk.

Similarly, there is rhythm in our breath with every inhalation and exhalation. When you are tense, your breath is shallow and the rhythm changes. Because your rhythm changes, your cells also begin to vibrate at a different frequency, which is similar to that of stress, thereby triggering cortisol (stress hormone) release.

During bedtime, when we are trying to slow down and put ourselves in a state of rest, our breathing rhythm changes and there is again a change in the way our cells vibrate. Cells sense this slowing down and thus vibrate in a way that puts us to sleep in relaxation mode.

Your pulse is a rhythm and so is your digestion. It is higher at certain times of the day and lower at certain times of the day. Circadian rhythm is all about sleep-wake cycles.

A woman's menstrual cycle is also a rhythm. Women experience it at a particular time of the month and there are changes in the frequency at which cells vibrate during this time, too. Brain waves also have a rhythm that carries a certain frequency. When we say something hurtful to someone, it is a change in frequency. The frequency of the listener's brain recognizes it and deciphers that this is something mean and hurtful.

Even what's keeping you engrossed in this book as you flip the pages is a specific frequency that you have tuned into. Now imagine someone shouting at you all of a sudden. Your frequency is immediately going to change and every single cell of your body is going to vibrate accordingly.

Your body has a tendency to heal itself naturally, provided immunity is strong, and that's possible only by taking one magic pill—lifestyle.

So everything, right from breathing to the menstrual cycle, has a particular rhythm designed by nature and we need to be in sync with these rhythms to remain healthy.

- If we are out of sync with our breathing, we feel anxious.

- If we are out of sync with our heart rate, we feel anxious; there's an increase in cortisol levels, inflammation, blood pressure and could lead to a heart attack.

- If we are out of sync with our digestion, we experience indigestion, gas, flatulence and acidity.

- If women are out of sync with their menstrual cycle, they experience weight-gain, facial-hair, mood swings and other side-effects.

The point, however, is that no drug, pill, medicine, or food can help recalibrate our desynchronized rhythms, except music.

Remember, every cell has a rhythm at which it vibrates. It can either be right or wrong. A cancer patient needs the rhythm of his cells to vibrate in the right way to successfully battle the disease. Vibrating at a frequency lower than where the patient is at the moment can actually make him feel sicker and possibly never recover. If a patient is sad, then that is a frequency he has created in every cell. The vibrational frequency of sad and negative emotions is very low. On the other hand, a patient who is positive has a higher frequency. This means each of us has the ability to change our rhythm and frequency by choosing the way we feel and also the kind of music we listen to. This is powerful because if a certain beat can change the frequency of a cell, then it can also change the frequency of an immune cell as well.

Did Allergies Exist in the Past?

Ask your grandparents. It is likely that when they were children, they probably had never heard about anyone being allergic to milk or to peanuts. And what about now? One can bet that you know someone allergic to gluten, dairy, or egg.

What is an allergy? It is an immune response of the body to a substance. Allergic reactions are on the rise and indeed they have been over the last few decades. There have been several attempts to explain the reasons why, but only recent research has been able to identify the crucial factor: microbiota. Your gut health determines your body's immune response towards food.

As we all know, 70 per cent of your immunity lies in the gut and hence gut microbiota are in charge of training the immune system. Issues start popping up when there are alterations in the composition of our gut microbiota. So how do you keep your gut clean and maintain a balance in microbiota?

Find your answers below:

Toxicity

When we reduce the amount of toxicity entering our body it leads to a healthy gut. A lot of things are not in our control, like pollution and food contamination, which is why we detoxify regularly. We help our body reduce a toxic overload through clean eating, regular detoxifying, fasting, a raw-till-lunch challenge, exercise, sweating, right quantity of water and probiotics.

Probiotics

We need probiotics on a daily basis. Now you can find it in kefir, fermented food items like idli, dosa, dhokla, etc. You can find it in certain types of yoghurt that contain live and active cultures. If you are a vegan, you can buy a great vegan probiotic, or you can make them at home, too.

Raw Food

The third thing we need is a portion of raw food (papaya, pineapple, mango, etc.) that provides digestive enzymes.

White Sugar

We need to be careful of the amount of white sugar we consume because it wipes out all of the good bacteria from your gut.

Caffeine

Excess caffeine creates inflammation in your gut. So, if you're consuming caffeine, make sure you drink sufficient water because it also acts as a diuretic.

Antibiotics

Control the use of antibiotics. They give you temporary relief and only treat your symptoms. Mother Nature has a lot to offer that can make you feel better. Start exploring because the damage that antibiotics cause is irreversible, and damages your gut.

Stress

Stress has a direct impact on your gut health, which is why you feel a churning or queasiness in your stomach when you're nervous about an activity. What are those butterflies in your stomach, then? They're nothing but your gut sending a communication to your brain and your gut communicates all the time. In fact, you have a second brain in your gut called your enteric nervous system (ENS). It is as real as your brain. So now think about all the cravings that you've been fighting. It could just be an unhealthy gut communicating with your brain in the wrong language.

Food for Every Season

When seasons change, have you ever wondered about doing something consciously to avoid falling sick? It's a sensitive time when a season changes; nature and our bodies adapt to this variation. That is when our immunity has to be strong and steady. There's a lot of disharmony between our reaction to the natural cycle due to our poor lifestyle and unhealthy eating. Suddenly staying healthy seems like an uphill task.

It is very important to consume seasonal foods and sync your body with the natural seasonal cycle. Eating seasonal foods also reinforces the balance between nature's resources and human health.

There is no lack of resources. In fact, nature is abundant and has provided us with everything as per our needs. With each changing season, nature offers an array of beautiful fresh products with high nutritional value.

Each season comes with its own set of naturally occurring food items. Foods grown in a particular season are perfectly designed to prepare our immunity. If we eat what grows in that particular season, we reduce our chances of falling sick.

There's a lot of significance attached to every seasonal food item. This whole cycle is so wonderfully outlined, every year in our country many crops are produced on the basis of seasons and have been a major source of livelihood and support for many local farmers.

Daily Activities to Keep You Healthy

Your palms contain pressure points that when activated help improve overall health. Some of these pressure points are for lungs, gall bladder, stomach, intestine, spleen, diaphragm, bladder and ovaries. Maintaining the health of these organs can also be attributed to daily chores like using a rolling pin to prepare rotis or preparing buttermilk using a hand blender. The rolling movements of these simple household appliances activate these pressure points.

Right Cookware

Cooking at home from scratch is one of the best ways to eat healthy. It allows you to control the quality of the ingredients and the cooking method. However, most of us ignore the utensils we use in the kitchen. You could be cooking a really healthy vegetable dish, but if you are cooking in low-quality pots or old non-stick pans, you are most likely doing more damage to your health. Using the wrong kind of utensils and cookware is one of the most potent causes of hormone disrupting chemicals, called endocrine-disrupting chemicals (EDCs). Over time, EDCs can set the stage for cancer, heart disease and cognitive damage.

Making the right cookware choices is an easy lifestyle change. Even the healthiest diet can result in health complications if your cookware is toxic.

Let's look at different cookware materials and their effects on health.

Aluminium Cookware

- Studies show that kitchen foil, cooking utensils and containers can contaminate your food with aluminium. This means that cooking with aluminium foil or cookware may increase the aluminium content in your diet.

- A study found that cooking with aluminium pots could exceed the daily aluminium limit, especially when cooking acidic foods. Researchers suggest that one should reduce the use of aluminium utensils and foil for cooking, especially if cooking with acidic foods, like tomatoes or lemons.

- Studies have suggested a link between aluminium and Alzheimer's.

- Research has shown that soluble aluminium salts can be absorbed from the stomach and the metal is deposited in the brain. Following the exposure to aluminium, aggregates of neurofilaments accumulate in the neurons. Aluminium influences a number of neuronal processes, such as increasing protein synthesis and neurotransmitter breakdown, to decreasing neurotransmitter reuptake and slow axonal transport.

- Studies have also linked aluminium to IBD and Crohn's disease as it has a harmful effect on intestinal inflammation and mucosal repair.

- A study concluded that aluminium cookware poses a greater danger to public health as compared to cast iron cookware.

Non-stick Cookware

- Most of the time, non-stick refers to a proprietary coating called Teflon.

- The non-stick properties of Teflon cookware are achieved with a coating of PTFE (polytetra-fluoroethylene), which is a plastic polymer that starts to leach toxins when heated above 300°C (572°F). These toxic fumes lead to flu-like symptoms called polymer fume fever, informally known as Teflon flu. A small number of case studies have also reported more serious side effects of exposure to overheated Teflon, including lung damage.

- Another chemical compound found in Teflon cookware is PFOA (perfluorooctanoic acid), which has been linked to a number of health conditions, including thyroid disorders, chronic kidney disease, liver disease and breast, prostate and ovarian cancer. It has also been linked to infertility and low birth weight.

- A 2007 study, conducted by the John Hopkins Bloomberg School of Public Health, showed alarming evidence that newborn infants face exposure to PFOA while in the womb. While PFOA can come from other sources, studies suggest the potential dangers of non-stick cookware.

The PFOA content is believed to be minimal in Teflon products, posing no risk to humans, but it is worth noting that many everyday objects contain this chemical compound. That's why it's best to limit your exposure wherever possible. Moreover, they are only safe to use while the coating is intact. This coating doesn't last too long and you should stop using the utensil once you notice any surface peeling and chipping.

Stainless Steel Cookware

- Stainless steel is a metal alloy that typically contains iron, chrome and nickel. It's called stainless because it is resistant to rust and corrosion, which makes it a great choice for cookware.

- Stainless steel tends to distribute heat evenly over its surface, making it especially great for griddle cooking and flat baking sheets.

- It is a mix of various metals, such as nickel and chromium that can migrate into food if your pan is damaged or worn but the amount is negligible and probably harmless unless you have certain allergies. Research suggests that people suffering from nickel allergy or skin rashes due to allergic contact dermatitis should not use stainless steel cookware.

- One must ensure that they buy 100 per cent food-grade stainless steel cookware.

Ceramic Cookware

- Steer clear of ceramic-coated, glazed, or decorated cookware. 100 per cent ceramic cookware is one of the best and safest options around since it's made with completely natural materials, isn't toxic, and won't chip or peel over time. The only downside is that 100 per cent ceramic can be pretty costly, but it will certainly last a long time.

- Glazes are applied to ceramics to give them strength and a smooth, shiny finish that prevents moisture from seeping into this non-metallic solid. Some of the ingredients used in making glazes include lead and cadmium that are toxic to human health. These heavy metals can leach out of the cookware and seep into the food.

- Ceramic-coated cookware is made of a metal such as aluminium that is coated with a hard film of polymer materials with a ceramic appearance. This coating contains binders, non-stick components, colour pigments and reinforcing agents.

- The soft ceramic coating isn't the most durable and begins to chip after several months of everyday use. Even when the coating is lead-free, chipped cookware can still present dangers as it's usually aluminium that's under the ceramic coating.

- For best results, ceramic cookware should be cleaned by hand rather than in the dishwasher. Most dishwasher detergents contain harsh chemicals that ruin the surface of ceramic cookware quickly. Second, the pressure of hot water sprayed on pans is hard on the pan's surface. Third, ceramic cookware tends to get scratched or chipped when coming into contact with other dishware.

Cast Iron Cookware

- Not only is cast iron known for its durability and even heat distribution, it is also one of the safest options out there because it doesn't contain any harmful chemicals that can leach into food.

- Unglazed cast iron can transfer notable amounts of iron into food, but unlike the metals that come off other types of pots and pans, iron is considered a healthy food additive by the Food and Drug Administration (USA).

- According to research, the introduction of iron pots for the preparation of food may be a promising innovative intervention for reducing iron deficiency and iron deficiency anaemia.

- If you're anaemic, eating food cooked in cast iron utensils can help improve your iron levels. But if you have haemochromatosis, a disorder that allows your body to absorb and maintain too much iron in your blood, you should avoid cast iron cookware.

- The non-stick quality of cast iron comes from seasoning. Seasoning is the term used for treating cast iron with oil and baking it. This fills in the porous surface of the cookware.

- Cast iron isn't difficult to clean since it requires a very specific method. Using soap to clean a cast iron utensil can ruin the seasoning. Use steel wool to clean the pan instead. Cast iron cookware is prone to gather rust if they're not dried properly. Dry with a towel, or heat on a stove for quick evaporation.

- Cast iron can be expensive, but it may be the only cookware ever needed as it lasts for decades.

Copper Cookware

- Copper cookware conducts heat well and has nutritional value due to its copper content. Usually, this kind of cookware has a base made of another metal like stainless steel with a copper coating.

- Like some other heavy metals, a small quantity of copper is very important for our bodies. Copper is responsible for the conversion of iron to haemoglobin, production of RBCs, cellular health, bone health, skin health, immunity, and also helps fight microbial infections. Adults need approximately 900 micrograms of copper per day, but an excess amount of it in the body can lead to heavy metal poisoning.

- Unlined copper isn't safe for everyday cooking as it can release copper when cooking, especially when cooking with citrus foods like tomatoes or something that has lemon, a staple ingredient in many Indian curries. And when it's coated, the coating often contains toxic elements like nickel or tin.

Glass

- Glass cookware is the most inert, meaning it will not leach chemicals, metals, or other harmful ingredients into your food. Tempered glass cookware can be used at high temperatures for baking and stovetop cooking.

- The only disadvantage is that glass utensils are very fragile. You should not continue using glass cookware that is chipped or cracked.

Silicone Cookware

- Most food-grade silicone utensils can withstand very high heat. However, certain silicone cookware can melt at very high temperatures and silicone liquid can seep into your food. If this happens, throw out the melted product and food. Don't use any silicone cookware at temperatures above 428°F (220°C).

- A study found that certain foods leach silicone into food. Silicone's safety at high temperatures has not been adequately tested. Most of the research into the impact of this synthetic material on health is in regard to silicone breast implants rather than food-related leaching. Until we have more proof, it is better to use silicone at low temperatures and in the refrigerator or freezer, but try to avoid it for high-temperature use.

- One should ensure they are buying utensils and bakeware made of 100 per cent food-grade silicone with zero plastic fillers. Pure silicone does not contain BPA (Bisphenol A). However, poorly made silicone bakeware and utensils that have fillers in them might contain BPA.

- One can do the twist test to check if the product contains fillers. Hold the silicone firmly between your fingers and twist. If the colour doesn't change, the product is filler-free. If the colour turns whitish, it contains fillers.

Plasticware

- Hot food in a plastic container can get contaminated leading to heart diseases, infertility, certain brain ailments, and even cancer. A Harvard research showed that BPA—found in certain types of plastics especially the kind used to make water bottles—plays a key role in weight gain.

- BPA, primarily found in a type of plastic called polycarbonate or PC, is toxic in large doses and can increase your risk of breast and prostate cancer and heart disease, among other health complications. Plasticware with BPA content is known to leach BPA into food when heated.

- Studies suggest consumers aren't off the hook buying BPA-free plastic. The results show that common BPA replacements—BPS, BPF, BPAF and diphenyl sulphone—are equally detrimental to health.

- Melamine resin is a tough plastic that can be found in children's dinner sets, many picnic sets and those noodle soup bowls you see on high rotation in food courts. Melamine too gives off toxic substances when it comes in contact with steaming hot food. Do not use melamine containers to heat food in a microwave (even if labelled microwave-safe). Researchers advise against using melamine containers or tableware for infants or children.

Chopping Board

- Most people use plastic chopping boards but even the best quality ones pose a health risk as chopping creates grooves that can harbour harmful microbes such as E. coli and salmonella. These germs find their way into cooked food via the next lot of sliced vegetables.

- Contamination is even more likely if the same board is used to chop meat or chicken. Some of these bugs are so stubborn that even cooking may not kill them. One should switch to wooden or rubber chopping boards and replace them every year.

Clay Pots

- Clay is healing for the human body. Ancient India used clay articles extensively, and it is one of the healthiest substances to use for cooking, eating and storing water.

- It's a natural way to cool water because earth and clay are porous in nature. In fact, water stored in clay matkas makes for one of the most refreshing drinks on a hot summer day. Add a few slices of lemon and organic jaggery and you end up having the perfect summer drink! Refrigerated water is great, but it can give you a sore throat. Drinking water out of clay pots is very satisfying because it helps you connect with nature. Since the earth is mineral-rich, a lot of beneficial minerals leach into water or the food that's cooked in clay ware.

- It's also a fantastic way to change the pH level of water, and it increases alkaline content. In fact, the pH level of water from a clay pot is higher than from a glass or plastic bottle.

- Clay is also loaded with microbes and vitamin B12 that is easily absorbed via skin and helps populate good gut bacteria and building colonies in the gut.

- One thing to note is that pure clay pots will turn moist on the outside signifying an unadulterated manufacturing process. Clay pots that don't leak have been lined and glazed and these varieties do not offer any health benefits.

- Clay is also used extensively for mud packs, face packs, and detoxifying masks for armpits since it helps draw out toxins from the lymphatic system.

- Clay pots are low-maintenance. All you need to do is empty their contents and leave them out in the sun for a couple of hours before reuse.

Safety Tips

Here are a few food safety tips for cooking with any kind of cookware. These tips will minimize your exposure to any metals or materials from your stove to your table.

- Don't store food in the pots or pans you've cooked in unless you're using glass or stone bakeware/cookware.

- Avoid using metal and hard cooking tools to stir food in your cookware as they can scratch and compromise the surface of your pots and pans.

- Minimize the amount of time your food is in contact with metals from pots and pans.

- Use a small amount of lubricants, such as ghee, olive oil or coconut oil, with any type of cookware to minimize the amount of invisible metal that sticks to your food.

- Clean pots and pans thoroughly after each use.

Conclusion

Material	Cookware	Drinkware	Utensils
Clay	√	√	√
Glass	√	√	√
Stainless Steel	√ (heating primarily)	√	√
Copper	×	√	×
Wood	×	√	√
Cast Iron	√	×	×
Plastic	×	×	×
Stone	√	×	√
Non-glazed Ceramic	√	√	√

Based on research, the safest cookware is that made of clay, ceramic, glass, cast iron, or stainless steel, especially higher quality products without contaminated glazing. Stay away from non-coated cookware that might leach heavy metals and other toxins into your food.

Traditional Wisdom of Including Certain Healthy Foods in Our Daily Life

Making yourself healthy is not a 'one-day' thing and if you are not including the practice in your daily routine, it will be hard to be consistent. Indians knew this very well and hence they included some healthy mixes in their daily life. These were not labelled as superfoods back then, but now they certainly are!

Turmeric Powder with Milk at Night

- Turmeric, or yellow gold, is a medicinal and culinary herb. Warm milk with a hint of turmeric was a common beverage in Indian households.

- Anti-inflammatory properties present in turmeric milk helps promote digestion, preventing stomach ulcers and diarrhoea.

- It's a potent anti-inflammatory, antioxidant, immunity-boosting, liver detoxifying, brain and neurological health-boosting spice. Curcumin, an active ingredient present in turmeric, is responsible for each of these benefits.

- One of the main benefits of turmeric milk is that it helps manage arthritic joint pains, body aches, muscle soreness, swollen joints, since it is capable of lowering inflammation levels.

- Good quality milk, on the other hand, is rich in tryptophan, an amino acid, that acts as a precursor to serotonin, a happy hormone that helps elevate our mood and puts us in a state of relaxation. Also, the presence of fat in milk aids better absorption of turmeric (curcumin) as this vital component is well absorbed in the presence of fat.

- This beverage is a great immunity and sleep enhancer. Studies show how turmeric has positive effects on brain degenerative conditions like Alzheimer's and Parkinson's. It lowers inflammation levels and can help you maintain supple and glowing skin in the long run (unless you are allergic to milk). If you are suffering from a cold and sore throat, then turmeric milk can also be your go-to option for quick relief and cure.

- Take it a step further and add a pinch of black pepper to this beverage to boost the bioavailability of curcumin. You could also add more spices like nutmeg and star anise.

- To reap maximum benefits from turmeric, make sure you consume the kind that is high in curcumin. Though there are a number of local varieties of turmeric available, a handful of them have consistent curcumin levels to deliver optimal benefits.

Note: Milk may not suit everyone, especially those with lactose intolerance. If you are fine having milk, it is advised to consume milk from Indian cow breeds (A2) that is free of hormones and antibiotics. If you are prone to excess mucus, then consume milk with caution.

Jaggery after Meals

Recent scientific studies have revealed the immense health benefits of jaggery (gur). Initially, it was referred to as 'the poor man's chocolate'. Jaggery is now considered an alternative to refined white sugar.

- Jaggery is a superfood during the winter season because it keeps the body warm.

- Jaggery is loaded with antioxidants and minerals such as zinc and selenium and helps boost low haemoglobin levels. Anaemia, or low haemoglobin levels, is a major concern among young women, teens and pregnant mothers in most parts of our country. A beverage of lemon water and jaggery is a great remedy to boost iron levels.

- The magnesium and potassium in jaggery helps dilate blood vessels, thereby aiding blood pressure management.

- Having a piece of jaggery right after meals can help improve digestion as jaggery stimulates the release of digestive enzymes. It can reduce gas and bloating.

- Additionally, it can also subdue your post-meal sugar cravings! Many places in northern India offer masala gur, a type of jaggery with spices like fennel, cumin and black pepper that further boost the digestion process.

- Jaggery acts as a mild laxative and can help alleviate constipation.

- It is rich in zinc and selenium, and in Ayurvedic practices, jaggery is also used as a detoxifying agent for the liver, and a blood purifier. It also supports detoxification of lungs to fight conditions like asthma, bronchitis and pneumonia. Mix 1 tsp of jaggery in warm water and have it as a natural treatment for cough and cold.

- It's a great cramp reliever for women going through PMS. A mix of 1 tsp jaggery and 1 tsp sesame seeds provides great relief in such cases.

- Jaggery and sugar have an equal impact on blood sugar

levels. Thus, it is important to consume them both in moderation to suit your individual health profile.

Having Some Form of Amla in Your Daily Diet

Indian gooseberry or amla is an inexpensive and easily available addition to your meals if you are looking to boost your immunity. Amla contains essential minerals and vitamins that are not only integral to our body's well-being, but also indispensable to preventing and managing some of the most common and widespread diseases.

- Amla combats common cold and cough due to its high vitamin C content.
- Vitamin C in amla aids synthesis of collagen that helps maintain the integrity and firmness of skin.
- Amla strengthens the inner walls of arteries often damaged due to exposure to pollution and faulty lifestyle habits like smoking.
- Indian gooseberry manages high levels of bad cholesterol and diabetes and reduces inflammation thanks to the presence of chromium, a trace mineral responsible for increasing insulin sensitivity of cells.
- Amla can be consumed in a variety of forms: juice, chutney, powder, pickle or murabba. Many people consume it along with jaggery. This can be beneficial, especially during winter.
- Amla is rich in vitamin C so people allergic to lemons can safely consume this as the next best alternative.

Chewing Tulsi Leaves

Tulsi (holy basil) is a sacred plant in Hindu belief. A tulsi plant is present in most Indian households as we worship the plant and use it for medicinal purposes.

- Holy basil is a known adaptogenic herb that helps address hormonal imbalances in the body.

- Tulsi works as a natural decongestant and immunity booster.

- It's a great stress relieving herb, and can be used as an alternative to tea and coffee.

- Slowly chewing a few leaves of tulsi will keep the stomach happy.

Fenugreek

- The green leafy vegetable is extremely rich in iron, folate, magnesium and chlorophyll.

- It can keep your cholesterol levels in check by reducing bad cholesterol (LDL and triglycerides), and maintaining heart health.

- It can also be used as a potent galactagogue for lactating mothers.

- It aids management of blood sugar levels in case of diabetes.

- Fenugreek (kasuri methi) is super-rich in fibre and promotes healthy bowel movement in case of constipation.

- Fenugreek has been used as a herb due to its medicinal properties and can be infused with coconut/castor/sesame oil for hair treatment. It has the capacity to halt or delay premature greying by retaining pigmentation.

- Fenugreek can easily become part of your diet since it is an ingredient in dals, vegetable gravies, pickles, chapattis, stir fries, dosas, chillas, etc. Though the spice is usually used as a flavouring agent, you can also use it as a mouth freshener after a meal.

- It is important to choose the right variant of kasuri methi to reap the most benefits.

Chyawanprash

Chyawanprash is an Ayurvedic superfood made up of nutrient-rich herbs and minerals. It is a *rasayana* formulation meant to restore the drained reserves of life force (*ojas*) and to preserve strength, stamina and vitality while stalling the course of ageing. The word 'chyawan' translates to degenerative change, and 'prasha' means an edible substance. The health benefits from major ingredients in chyawanprash are stated in the table below:

Common Name	Therapeutic Role
Vasaka, arusa (Malabar nut)	Helps soothe ulcers, expectorant, bronchodilator, anti-allergic, bile stimulatory, cardiovascular and respiratory disorders
Bael	Helps heal gut lining
Agaru, akil	Helps alleviate asthma, reduces general body pain; anti-inflammatory and antimicrobial
Banslochan	Helps improve menstrual flow and is also an aphrodisiac
Punarnawa, gadahapurna, gadah bindo	Excellent antioxidant, diuretic, anti-inflammatory, and helps reduce fever
Tejpat, tejpatra	Helps soothe ulcers and improves liver health
Dalchini	Good for liver and gut

Kachur, ban haldi, narkachur	Reduces bloating, and alleviates diarrhoea
Nagarmotha, mustak, musta	Relieves pain, improves bone health, good for the gut and liver
Shalparni, sarivan	Reduces fatigue, improves lung, heart and brain health
Elaichi	Helps treat nausea, heartburn and intestinal spasms
Amalaki, amla	Helps improve immunity, nervous system, liver health, heart health, memory, longevity, etc.
Gambhari, gamhar, kashmarya	Great to improve strength
Pushkarmul	Excellent for respiratory health (asthmatics)
Jivanti	Arrests abnormal cell growth and improves vision, immunity and life expectancy
Ulat kanta	Boosts iron and improves liver and gut health
Nagakesar	Relieves urinary tract disorders, gout and swelling
Sahasrapatra, neelkamal	Calming and nourishing, it promotes strength and relieves excessive bleeding disorders
Aralu, bhut-vriksha, shyonak	Improves well-being by improving the nervous system, heart health, and is a great energizer
Mudgaparni	Improves semen and sperm quantity; is an aphrodisiac

Bhumyamalaki, bhumi amla	Antioxidant, laxative, improves bile secretion, antiviral
Pippali	Helps relieve cough, respiratory infections and hepatitis
Kakdasinghi	Improves bile secretion, a bronchodilator, expectorant, carminative
Arni, agnimanth	Laxative, relieves cold and improves digestion
Raktachandan	Tonic, helps improve blood sugar levels, aphrodisiac, reduces fever, soothes respiratory tract
Til taila	Anti-inflammatory, improves wound healing
Bala, bariyara	Improves heart health, aphrodisiac, strength/vitality promoter
Brihati, bari kateri, vanbhanta	Prevents formation of gas in the gastrointestinal tract
Kantakaari, chotikateri	Helps relieve flu and helps in dilation of lungs
Paatla	Anti-inflammatory, improves iron and helps in purifying blood
Mashaparni	Improves vigour and virility, aphrodisiac, energizes the body
Harad, haritaki	Appetite stimulant, improves central nervous system
Guduchi, chinnodbhava	Apoptogenic, helps protect cells
Gokhru, gokshur	Aphrodisiac, elevates mood, diuretic and cardiotonic

Prishnaparni, pithawan	Improves energy levels
Draksha, munakka	Helps in relieving irritation, is an aphrodisiac, diuretic, relieves constipation, cures thirst, good for asthma patients
Go ghrita	Improves overall physical and mental strength
Madhu	Immunomodulator, wound healing, antioxidant, anti-ageing relieves cough and cold, antiseptic, sore throat, helps soothe ulcers
Shatavari, shatavar	Adaptogenic, galactagogue, helps soothe ulcers; an antioxidant, good for the eyes
Varahikand, varahi	Aphrodisiac, helps soothe ulcers, and improves strength
Vidaarikand	Aphrodisiac, antioxidant, galactagogue, nervine tonic, increases mental stability and increases sperm count
Ashwagandha, asgandh	Aphrodisiac, adaptogenic, antioxidant, promotes strength
Abhraka bhasma	Cell regeneration, improves mental stability, useful in digestive impairment, malabsorption syndrome, asthma and cough
Shukti bhasma	Relieves heartburn, reduces allergic symptoms, improves bone health
Shringa bhasma	Expectorant, reduces inflammation of lungs and chest cavity

| Makardhawaja | Helps cure male impotency, erectile dysfunction, and premature ejaculation. It is also good for heart health. |
| Laung | Has a pleasant aroma and is anti-inflammatory |

All these ingredients may not be easily available. Here is the recipe with optimal health benefits:

Ingredients:

- 2–3 cups amla (Indian gooseberry)
- 1 cup organic jaggery
- 5 to 6 tbsp A2 ghee
- Spice mixture to be ground
- 6–8 elaichis (green cardamom)
- 1 tbsp whole black pepper
- 5 gm nutmeg
- 1 bay leaf
- 1-inch cardamom stick
- 1–2 tbsp saunf (fennel seeds)
- 5 gm cloves
- 5–6 strands kesar (saffron)
- 10 gm dry ginger powder

Method:

- Wash amlas and pat them dry.
- Add water and amlas to a pressure pan and close the lid. Boil the amlas for 2 whistles or 10 minutes on full pressure.

- Turn the flame off and let it sit in steam until the pressure is released.
- Drain the water; easily remove pits from the boiled amlas.
- Add pulp in a blender and make a smooth puree with a spoonful of water to ease grinding.
- Add some ghee in a pan and mix amla puree.
- Keep sautéing for 10 minutes until ghee separates from the amla puree.
- Add jaggery powder to the amla puree.
- Keep sautéing till you achieve a thick, sticky mass.
- On the side, take ingredients of the spice mixture and blend finely.
- Add ground spice mixture to the pan and mix well.
- Continue to cook for another 5 minutes till everything is well combined.
- Let it cool down and transfer to an airtight jar.

Consume 1 spoon of chyawanprash daily to build immunity. Children can take 1 tbsp added to milk.

Notes:

- The dry spice mixture can be added to your tea to enhance flavour.
- The amla–jaggery mixture is used as a jam too to spread on roti, paratha, etc.
- Once stored in an airtight container, chyawanprash has a shelf life of 4 months.
- Amla, the base ingredient in chyawanprash, detoxifies the body and cleanses the blood, liver, spleen and lungs. It tones the body and enhances youthfulness and promotes healthy muscle and mass.

- Dry ginger powder is anti-inflammatory and helps relieve cold.
- Cinnamon has carminative and astringent properties.
- Nutmeg has antibacterial properties.
- Black pepper helps increase the production of hydrochloric acid that the stomach needs for digestion.
- Saffron has antioxidant and antidepressant properties.
- Chyawanprash is an Ayurvedic superfood. It strengthens the immune system and revitalizes the psychosomatic system.

Indian Superfoods

Mango

During the onset of summers, my mailbox is flooded with innumerable questions about one particular fruit. 'Can I eat mangoes if I have diabetes?' 'Wouldn't mangoes raise my sugar levels?'. 'Oh! Mangoes are too much sugar. Am I going to put on weight if I eat mangoes?'

Before we get into understanding how healthy a mango actually is, let's get one thing straight. You shouldn't be scared of anything that grows naturally. No edible fruit provided by nature can be unhealthy for us. Instead, you should be scared of everything that's packaged and processed. You should be scared of living a poor and sedentary lifestyle. You should be scared of overeating mangoes because overeating anything (even a fruit) creates a spike in our blood sugar levels. You should be scared of the endless medication you pop—not a fruit.

1. Mango is an extremely healthy fruit for everyone, including a diabetic. It's one of the richest sources of vitamin C, A, E, K and most B vitamins (except B12). It contains traces of omega-3 and omega-6 fatty acids and is loaded with minerals and fibre. One ripe mango provides approximately 29–32 gm of sugar which is a fruit sugar and a glycaemic load of 10.

2. There is no point eyeing a mango warily. If you choose to eat a bowl of mango chunks, an entire mango or half a mango, it's always best to include a few nuts and seeds during or after the fruit. Mango is a fibre-rich fruit and your sugar levels will not spike if eaten in moderation.

3. Mangoes also contain a substance called mangiferin that has an anti-viral and anti-inflammatory impact on our body, and also has the capacity to affect certain enzymes in our body that play an important role in blood sugar management. So, there is really no connection between a mango and diabetes just because the fruit has a natural tendency to raise blood sugar levels. Additionally, mangiferin also has the ability to loosen and remove fatty deposits from our liver.

4. Most locals and Goans believe that mangoes grow at this particular time of the year because of the beauty and wisdom of nature. Mangoes are a summer fruit because they tend to have a cooling impact on the body. That's why one must stick to eating local and seasonal produce always.

5. There are many people who associate mangoes with skin breakouts and heat boils. The truth is that if you have toxins in your body and eat mangoes, the detoxification process will leads to skin breakouts. This is similar to eliminating toxins from the body in the form of pimples and boils. It is our body's way of releasing heat and toxins in the form of pus. Unfortunately, we react instead of responding and trying to understand the inner workings of our bodies.

6. Another thing to note about the king of fruits is the abundance of vitamin C, a powerful antioxidant and immunity-boosting vitamin. Our bodies are incapable of manufacturing vitamin C, hence we rely on fruits, vegetables, nuts and seeds to fulfil our daily requirement.

Adults aged 19 to 64 need 40mg of vitamin C a day. Vitamin C tends to have a positive impact on weight management and sugar levels. It has the capacity to flush out fatty acids from our blood.

7. We see a drop in immunity just after the monsoon. Mangoes flourish just before the monsoon sets in so that we can boost our immunity against monsoon-related sicknesses. This helps in a healthy transition from one season to another. Most locals in Goa and the coastal regions believe this and it makes complete sense.

8. Nature has an inbuilt mechanism of preparing everyone for the next season. The odds of you falling ill are drastically reduced if you eat what grows during a particular season/region. There are people who eat 5–6 mangoes a day. Now, that's certainly overdoing it. There is a whole season lying in front of you to enjoy this divine fruit. Eat one a day or maybe two. If your diabetes is at a very advanced stage, you may want to have half a mango in the morning and enjoy the other half in the evening, along with nuts and seeds if your sugar levels tend to rise quickly. Also remember, mangoes contain negligible amounts of fat and have nothing to do with weight gain.

There is so much goodness packed into a mango that we can blindly trust the goodness of nature's edible gifts.

Amla

1. Mix 1 tbsp of amla juice with 1 tsp unpasteurized honey and 1 tsp ginger juice to treat sore throat and cold.

2. Amla enhances immunity by increasing the white blood cell count in the body.

3. 30 ml amla juice can detoxify your liver and help with digestion.

4. Suck a piece of amla to improve appetite.

5. For thick, dark hair, you can eat fresh amla every day or apply its paste to the hair roots. When amla is no longer in season, make a paste of amla powder with water and apply to the roots.

6. Amla acts as a blood purifier that helps control acne, blemishes and various skin problems. Moreover, amla acts as a purifier that helps cleanse the pores, remove dead cells and tightens the skin, and delays wrinkles, tired face, etc.

7. Studies show that drinking amla juice with honey is great for the eyes.

8. Amla acts as a herbal therapy for strengthening bones due to the fact that it lowers osteoclasts. Osteoclasts are the cells that absorb bone tissue during growth and healing. Indian gooseberry helps with calcium absorption that is most essential for bone health.

9. Minerals and nutritional vitamins in amla help reduce menstrual cramps.

10. Taking 1 tbsp of amla juice improves the quality of sleep.

11. Amla is a tonic for the heart. It helps strengthen coronary heart muscle tissues thereby improving the pumping of blood. Amla consists of potassium that reduces stress in arteries and blood vessels.

12. Amla improves respiratory issues like allergies, asthma, bronchitis, chronic cough, etc.

13. Take 1 tbsp amla juice with honey thrice a day to treat dry cough.

14. Amla helps overcome paralytic problems.

15. Amla naturally controls blood sugar levels and LDL cholesterol. To improve benefits, take amla juice (10–15 ml) with aloe vera juice regularly.

16. Amla juice improves metabolism and helps with weight loss. It also flushes toxins from the body.

17. Amla is recommended to limit swelling or inflammation. Consequently, amla can help with arthritis, pancreatitis and age-related renal ailments.

In brief, Indian gooseberry is a great natural medicinal drug for a wide range of health disorders. You should consume amla during winters when it is readily available, and its powdered form can work during the rest of the year.

Banana

Bananas have many medicinal properties. It has tryptophan, an amino acid that plays a vital role in boosting and retaining memory.

Its fundamental health benefits are:

1. Banana is rich in potassium and very low in sodium. These vital components help regulate blood pressure. The high potassium content helps improve heart rhythm.

2. Nutrients like fibre, vitamin C and B-6 are also good for coronary heart health.

3. Because of its predominant components, potassium and magnesium, bananas help reduce headaches. Make a paste of banana peel and apply it on your forehead to reduce headaches within seconds.

4. Bananas help get rid of teeth discolouration, whitens enamel and improves your smile. Its magnesium and potassium content helps clear yellowish stains and protects teeth cavities. You can whiten your enamel by rubbing the inside of the peel on your teeth for a minute or two every day.

5. To reduce wrinkles, rub the inside of the peel on your

face and leave it for thirty minutes. Then wash your face with clean water.

6. For jaundice, consume banana with honey twice a day.

7. Bananas are good for those suffering from diarrhoea, when electrolytes like potassium are depleted and weakness sets in. It can be given to small children, too. Mash a banana, add some mishri powder and give it to your child. Repeat it 3–4 times a day.

8. Bananas can reduce acidity and heartburn. Chop it into small pieces and combine it with yoghurt. It also helps relieve flatulence and reduce bloating.

9. Banana helps with fat loss due to soluble fibre. This soluble fibre helps slow down the digestive process, and keeps hunger pangs at bay. Add bananas with milk to your diet if you want to lose weight.

10. The inside of a banana peel can help alleviate the sharp pain caused by a bee sting.

11. Grinding the peel in a mixer into a paste and applying it to your face can help with pimples.

12. In case of warts, rub the inside of a banana peel on the affected area every day for 2–3 minutes, and apply peel paste at night. The warts will disappear completely after a few days.

13. Banana has tryptophan amino acid which produces the serotonin hormone. This hormone performs a necessary function of controlling temper and depression.

14. Bananas are beneficial in increasing white blood cell count.

15. The potassium in bananas enhances muscular tissues by controlling cramps. Eating 1–2 bananas daily as part of your exercise regimen helps preserve energy during exercising because it provides a healthy supply of carbohydrates.

16. Bananas comprise tryptophan, potassium and magnesium that are muscle relaxants. Therefore, eat one before sunset, it will make you sleep well at night.

17. The fibre content of bananas is great for the digestive system and natural digestion of meals.

18. The antacid properties of a banana provides relief from stomach ulcers.

19. Bananas have deworming properties that help kill intestinal worms and dispose of them through excretion.

20. Bananas keep bones healthy.

21. Bananas are a source of vitamin C that preserves the immune system.

22. If you are slim and want to gain weight, the banana is an excellent solution. Eat it with milk twice a day in addition to other food.

23. Banana controls cholesterol, reduces blood clots, and thins the blood due to its potassium content.

24. If your baby has swallowed a coin, get him/her a ripe banana. The object will be excreted.

25. If you have a swelling on any part of your body, apply banana pulp with wheat flour. Mash 1 or 2 bananas (as per requirement) and add some wheat flour to make dough. Then heat the mixture, transfer to a cloth and apply it to the affected area.

26. Banana has amino acids that reduce anxiety hormones in the body. Therefore, eat bananas to eliminate tension.

27. Mashed banana with ghee can help with a frequent urination problem.

28. 1 banana with curd made from A2 milk can treat mouth ulcers.

29. If you are suffering from drastic hair fall, mash the pulp of 1 or 2 bananas and add the juice of 1 lemon. Apply

the paste on your hair. Leave it on for 10–15 minutes and wash with clean water.

30. Banana pulp with honey (2–3 tbsp) can act as a moisturizer for dry and hard hair.

31. Banana pulp eliminates lifeless cells and makes your pores and skin tender and shiny. Mix 1 tbsp of sandalwood powder and ½ tbsp of honey with the pulp of a banana and apply the paste on your face. Leave it for 20–25 minutes and wash with water.

Bael/Wood Apple

1. Gastric ulcers occur due to an imbalance in the acidic levels in the stomach. Wood apple consists of phenolic compounds (antioxidants) that help deal with gastric ulcers. Actually, the internal lining is broken due to long-standing acidity in the belly that forms ulcers. Bael also reduces acidity.

2. Bael leaves are scientifically proven to have hypoglycaemic and antioxidant properties. Extracts from these leaves offer energy to the pancreas that corrects the insulin degree continuously and consequently helps control blood sugar levels. Simply bite/chew 4–5 wood apple leaves every morning on an empty stomach, or extract and consume its juice. To extract the juice, grind 8–10 leaves and 4–5 black peppercorns with a little water in a blender. For better results, add tulsi leaves to the mix.

3. Bael leaves help decrease blood cholesterol; chew 4–5 bael leaves, or consume one spoonful of bael leaf juice on an empty stomach. To extract juice from the leaves, grind a few leaves in a mortar and extract the juice with a thin cotton cloth.

4. The unripe or half-ripe fruit can alleviate chronic diarrhoea. Mix bael pulp or powder with jaggery for best results.

5. Because of its laxative properties, ripe bael fruit can also be used to treat constipation. Consuming bael on a regular basis for 2–3 months will help clean your intestine and reduce constipation. To cure hard stool, soak 3 spoons of bael fruit pulp with 1 spoon tamarind in a cup for 2 hours. Then, mash it with fingertips and strain; add some mishri before consuming.

6. It's a summer coolant.

7. The pulp of the fruit mixed with ghee acts as a heart tonic.

8. Wood apple helps improve intestinal activity and can be used to treat piles. The unripe fruit is a remedy for piles and haemorrhoids. Prepare a decoction of bael fruit pulp with some fennel seeds and ginger; consume lukewarm with honey.

9. Bael consists of beta-carotene, thiamine and riboflavin that help remove liver problems. The regular consumption of bael prevents harmful toxins from affecting the liver.

10. Regular consumption of bael improves kidney power and therefore helps overcome urinary diseases.

11. Murabba of bael fruit can alleviate dysentery. Mix dry bael powder and coriander powder (½ spoon each) with 1 tsp of mishri and consume with water twice daily.

12. Bael decoction can treat blood in urine and stool. Collect dry bael powder, fennel seeds powder (3 tsp each), and dry ginger powder (2 tsp); add all three in a glass of water. Boil in a pan until the liquid has reduced to half its amount. Now strain and consume while lukewarm, twice a day.

13. Scurvy results from vitamin C deficiency. Bael contains high amounts of vitamin C that may additionally help protect from pores and skin sicknesses.

14. Due to its antimicrobial, anti-viral and anti-fungal properties, bael treats quite a number of infections in the body.

15. Make a pack with aloe vera and apply on your face for glowing skin. Combine wood apple extract with honey, aloe vera, sandalwood powder and rose water in a bowl and apply on the face for 25–30 minutes.

16. Bael is an excellent remedy for leucoderma or vitiligo. White spotting can lighten over time with the topical use of bael.

17. Since bael is rich in vitamins, it can benefit your hair and treat scalp problems. Mix bael fruit extract with coconut oil and almond oil and apply this combination on your hair and scalp.

18. The juice of bael leaves with honey can help control fever.

19. Wood apple bark may additionally be used to treat malaria.

20. Bael juice enhances breast milk production.

21. Bael fruit is a good diuretic that works as a blood cleanser.

22. Bael is anti-inflammatory in nature; use its extracts on the exposed region to reduce inflammation. A warm poultice of the leaves reduces inflammation.

Ajwain/Carom

1. Chew 1 tsp of ajwain 2–3 times daily to treat common cold.

2. Simply ingest a paste of carom seeds, honey and rock salt to cure cough.

3. Use ajwain water in an earthen pot or its concoction to cure high fever. Add 4 cups of water in an earthen pot

and soak 24 gm carom seeds early in the morning. Keep it in the shade for a day. Strain and drink this water next morning. This has been known to cure fever that has been plaguing the patient for 10 to 12 days.

4. One can reduce malaise or general discomfort with a combination of ajwain and cinnamon (½ tsp each).

5. Ajwain contains active enzymes that help facilitate the release of gastric juices. It boosts our digestive machinery. Therefore, chewing on a small quantity of carom seeds after a meal like mouth freshener is a good idea.

6. Grind carom seeds into a paste and apply on the affected area for temporary relief from a scorpion bite.

7. Consume ajwain water from an earthen pot for 10–12 days to reduce intestinal inflammation.

8. Consume half or one tsp of ajwain with lukewarm water, 3–4 times a day to reduce throat inflammation.

9. Carom seed oil has antibiotic and anaesthetic properties that make it excellent for limiting musculoskeletal swelling and pain. To prepare this oil, add carom seeds, garlic cloves and asafoetida in mustard oil and boil thoroughly. Let it cool and store in a jar after straining/sieving, for use whenever required. Always apply this oil slightly lukewarm to the affected area.

10. Combine one spoon of carom seed powder in some radish juice and take it for 2–3 weeks. It breaks kidney stones into smaller portions and flushes them out.

11. Apply carom oil 3–4 times daily to treat toenail fungal infection.

12. Massage your hair regularly with a mix of carom and coconut oil to improve hair growth.

13. Carom seeds have anti-fungal and antioxidant properties. If you suffer from a skin disorder, a thick

paste of ajwain can be applied on the affected area 3–4 times daily.

14. If your head is covered with tiny pink boils, apply a paste of carom seeds with lemon juice.

15. For zits/skin spots, use ajwain paste with curd. Make a paste of 20 gm carom seeds with 25 gm curd and apply this mix on your face; wash your face with lukewarm water after a while.

16. Ajwain is good for deworming kids. Mix ½ tsp roasted ajwain powder with 1 tsp jaggery powder and give this mixture at bedtime for 3 days.

17. Steam inhalation/hot and dry fermentation of carom seeds is excellent for reducing chest congestion and releasing mucus. Congestion can be eliminated by inhaling the scent or fumes of ajwain. For this, you have to warm some ajwain on a pre-heated hot pan (tawa) and breathe in the fumes.

18. Drink ajwain tea for sore throat.

19. A small quantity of carom seeds can help reduce acidity.

20. Carom seeds help burn fat by increasing metabolism. A mixture of ajwain, fenugreek seeds and black cumin seeds helps with fat loss.

21. To reduce insomnia, drink a cup of ajwain water 1½–2 hours prior to before retiring for the night.

22. Asthma patients can find some relief by ingesting roasted ajwain and jaggery (5 gm) with lukewarm water.

23. To relieve congestion in kids, make a swag of lightly roasted ajwain, and bundle into a soft cotton cloth. Use as a fomentation on the child's chest. Hold the swag near the nostrils to eliminate nasal congestion.

24. Carom seed is a natural painkiller that offers relief from all types of toothache.

25. One drop of carom seed oil can even limit extreme earache.

26. Ajwain oil is good for gout and arthritis pain.

27. You can apply a beaten paste of carom seeds externally on the stomach of a baby to relieve colic pain.

28. If your infant is crying restlessly and a doctor is not available immediately, you can try ajwain for instant relief. Boil ½ tsp of ajwain in 1500 ml of water on a low flame for 5–10 minutes. Let it cool and serve a few spoonfuls to your infant to treat colic pain.

29. Prepare a concoction of fennel seeds and ajwain. Boil ½ tsp fennel seeds with ½ tsp of carom seeds in 2 litres of water on low flame for 10 minutes; let it cool. Then serve a few spoonfuls of this concoction to your toddler to cure gas and colic pain.

30. Carom seeds contain thymol that is antispasmodic and can reduce stomach cramps. Mix a few drops of ajwain oil with a tbsp of coconut oil and apply on your lower abdomen.

31. For menstrual stomach ache, simply boil 1 tsp of carom seeds in drinking water and consume. It relaxes the uterus and alleviates discomfort.

32. You can use soaked carom seeds for irregular menses.

33. Carom seed helps increase libido. It works as a stimulant or a natural aphrodisiac to make you sexually active. Simply bite a few carom seeds after dinner before going to bed at night. Or use carom seeds with tamarind and ghee to increase libido.

34. Ajwain can help minimize premature ejaculation. Roast some ajwain and tamarind kernels with ghee in a pan. After roasting, grind into a paste. Now mix 1 tsp of this paste in a glass of hot milk with 1 tbsp of honey and drink regularly before bedtime.

35. Ingest carom seeds soaked in lemon juice to treat impotency.

36. Eczema is a condition that makes your skin red, itchy, cracked and inflamed. Carom seeds are good to heal these patches of eczema. At first, wash the patches with carom seed water. Boil 1 tsp of carom seeds in 500 ml water for 10 minutes; let it cool. Grind some carom seeds to make a paste with lukewarm water. Now apply this paste on the affected place 2–3 times a day.

37. Use ajwain with curry leaves and raisins to delay premature greying.

38. Carom seeds with neem leaves or carom seeds with fenugreek seeds can help diabetics maintain a healthy lifestyle.

39. 25 gm ajwain, 50 gm black sesame seeds, 100 gm jaggery; roast carom seeds and black sesame seeds separately; grind all three and combine well. 1 tsp of this mixture, twice a day for 2–3 weeks, can help reduce bed-wetting.

40. Polyuria, or excessive passing of urine, can be treated by drinking a mixture of carom seeds (1 tsp) with bael leaf juice (20 ml), twice daily. You can ingest ajwain with sesame seeds, (half a tsp each), with water twice a day to control urination.

41. Roast carom seeds and fennel seeds in equal proportion and consume them post meals like mouth freshener, to increase milk production.

42. Carom seeds with buttermilk can help treat piles and bleeding.

43. Alcohol craving, or dipsomania, can be kept at bay by chewing roasted ajwain.

44. Ajwain tea reduces inflammation in gut, thus helping with gastritis.

45. Soak carom seeds (½ tsp) in a cup of water for 3–4 hours and consume every day after sieving to treat paralysis.

46. Ajwain tea purifies your blood. It improves blood circulation and limit pores and skin conditions.

47. To cure any kind of gum problem, roast carom seeds and grind into a fine powder. Brush your teeth with this powder regularly.

Karela/Bitter Gourd Juice

1. Bitter gourd (or bitter melon) is frequently used as a remedy for diabetes. It has been found that bitter gourd or karela has unique phyto-constituents known as charantin and polypeptide-P that have been proved to have hypoglycaemic and insulin-like effects. That's why it helps lower the blood sugar level specifically in Type 2 diabetes. Ingest 10–20 ml juice on an empty belly every day to control blood sugar.

2. Karela has blood-purifying qualities and is great for pores and skin problems.

3. Urine retention is a common issue among older people and bitter gourd leaves help improve urine retention.

4. Karela works as a liver tonic if consumed regularly. 20 gm bitter gourd juice, 5 gm mustard powder, 3 gm rock salt powder; mix all and consume on an empty stomach.

5. Extract the juice of bitter gourd and rub your soles for 5–10 minutes before going to bed at night to alleviate burning sensation.

6. Bitter gourd is a natural supply of vitamin K. It has anti-inflammatory properties and is good for arthritis and gout patients. Bitter gourd paste can eliminate infection/inflammation.

7. Apply the paste on your neck and cover it with a cotton fabric to reduce throat swelling. This can be highly beneficial for thyroid patients.

8. Karela juice with asafoetida kills stomach worms and acts as a deworming agent.

9. Bitter gourd juice stimulates the liver and aids the secretion of bile juices that is crucial for metabolism, thereby aiding fat loss.

10. Drink 10–15 ml fresh bitter gourd juice daily to get rid of skin infections.

11. Karela juice also works against kidney stones.

12. Bitter gourd is rich in vitamin B1, B2, B3, C, A, folic acid, zinc, manganese and a host of other nutrients. It is high in beta-carotene that helps prevent vision-associated problems such as eye infection and cataract, and is also known to improve eyesight.

13. Bitter gourd contains a lot of fibre that makes the stool softer and relieves constipation. The juice can have the same effect, as well.

Clove

1. Clove is a natural pain killer, especially for toothache. Simply, take one clove and put it on the affected tooth for sometime.

2. In addition to that, clove oil, eugenol, works as an antiseptic and pain reliever. It works as a local anaesthetic and antiseptic for teeth and gums.

3. Chewing on a clove can control bad breath.

4. Boil a clove in water and gargle 2–3 times a day for good oral health.

5. Take some coconut oil in a bowl, mix 8–10 drops of clove oil, and massage your head for pain alleviation.

6. Dab 2–3 drops of clove oil in a cotton handkerchief and keep sniffing to clear a blocked nose.

7. Boil 4–5 cloves in a cup of water and drink thrice a day to relieve cold.

8. Ingest a pinch of clove powder with honey 2–3 times a day to relieve chronic cough.

9. Cloves are the richest source of antioxidants such as anthocyanins and quercetin. If you eat one clove with green cardamom daily after your meals, it will help remove toxins from the body.

10. Clove also contains a variety of flavonoids. Its oil has anti-inflammatory properties that help reduce inflammation of joints and in controlling pain. Add one spoon of clove oil in 2–3 spoons of coconut or sesame oil. Massage the joints gently whenever you have swelling and pain.

11. Grind some cloves to make a paste and apply this on the aching joint to treat arthritis and rheumatism.

12. Clove provides relief from a sore throat because of its essential oil, eugenol. Boil some water in a pan and add 2–3 drops of clove oil. Inhale the steam after covering your head with a towel.

13. To control vomiting, take a pinch of clove powder, add some honey and swallow.

14. Clove oil is used as a mental refresher tonic. Rub some drops on your forehead to release stress and mental fatigue.

15. You can make a flavoured tea by adding clove, mint, basil and green cardamom in water. Boil and drink with honey to release stress and mental fatigue.

16. If you're dealing with work stress, apply only one drop of clove oil on your wrist. At the same time, rub one drop of clove oil with some olive oil on your forehead, too. It will help you sleep better.

17. Whenever you feel a build-up of stomach gas, boil half a glass of water and add two powdered cloves. Cool and drink.

18. Cloves are used in various home remedies to treat different digestive problems such as diarrhoea, nausea, indigestion, etc. In such cases, boil half a glass of water with cloves (powder of 2 pods), add a pinch of hing, cool and drink.

19. Grind two pods of clove and mix with 100 ml water. Mix a little mishri powder and consume to reduce heartburn.

20. Clove oil mixed with mustard oil will provide relief from earache.

21. Boil 5–6 cloves in half cup of water on low heat. Let it cool and drink lukewarm with 1 spoon of honey for asthma relief.

22. To treat muscle cramps, apply 1–2 ml clove oil with an equal quantity of vinegar on the affected area.

23. Clove is a good disinfectant for an eye stye. Grind a few cloves and add some water. Add this paste on the stye and leave it to dry for a few hours.

24. By applying clove oil directly on the affected areas, you can remove acne, scars and blemishes. Since clove oil is quite strong, dilute it by mixing with multani mitti or aloe vera gel.

25. One drop of clove oil on the wrist of a pregnant woman can help her keep morning sickness at bay. Apply 1–2 drops of clove oil on a cotton cloth or handkerchief to inhale.

26. Mix 1–2 clove oil drops in some aloe vera gel or olive oil and massage your face gently to keep wrinkles away.

Cucumber Juice

1. Half a glass of cucumber juice in the morning can help with any urine retention or urine passing issues. Cucumber is 95 per cent water; it keeps you hydrated and helps the body eliminate toxins.

2. Have half a glass of cucumber juice twice a day, in the morning and evening, to cure frequent urination.

3. Drink a glass of cucumber juice with black salt and lemon juice to cure yellow urination.

4. 250 ml of cucumber juice, three times a day, helps remove kidney stones.

5. Cucumber contains trypsin, an enzyme that helps digest protein. By including cucumber in your daily diet, you can control constipation, too. A cucumber and tomato salad with black salt powder, black pepper powder and lemon juice improves digestion.

6. Cucumber contains potassium that is very healthy for high blood pressure patients.

7. Cucumber is good for bone health since it contains vitamin K that is vital for improving bone density. It is a good source of silica that helps in the construction of connective tissues like bones, ligaments, muscles, cartilage and tendons in our body. A mixture of cucumber and carrot juice is beneficial for rheumatic conditions.

8. Cucumber juice also helps flush out uric acid.

9. Cucumber juice is most effective for hair growth because of its silicon and sulphur content. After washing your hair with shampoo, rinse it again with cucumber juice to make it shinier and stronger.

10. For stronger hair, drink cucumber juice with carrot, spinach or lettuce.

11. Cucumber helps pancreatic cells produce insulin, making it a good choice for diabetic patients.

12. Cucumber, an alkaline food, helps regulate pH levels and neutralize acidity.

13. Joint pain or arthritis is a common health problem and cucumber is good for bone health. When taken along with carrots, cucumber alleviates joint pain and arthritis.

14. Cucumber is good for skin problems because of vitamin C and antioxidants. For curing facial black patches and brown spots on the face, apply cucumber pieces on the affected area for thirty minutes, twice a day; it will cure patches within one month.

15. To treat sunburns, rub cucumber juice with turmeric on the affected area 2–3 times in a day.

16. Cucumber is the best therapy for tired eyes. The fatigue that sets in after staring at a screen for long hours can be cured by putting cucumber slices on your eyes for ten minutes.

17. One cucumber a day can provide relief from periodontitis.

18. Cucumber is rich in soluble fibre; it reduces hunger pangs and stops you from overeating.

Elaichi/Cardamom

1. To clear a sore throat, chew 1–2 green cardamom pods on an empty stomach in the morning and at night, and drink lukewarm water.

2. Cardamom has anti-inflammatory properties that help reduce throat inflammation. Green cardamom paste with some radish juice is known to cure swelling of the throat glands.

3. As certain studies have revealed, the antimicrobial and antibacterial properties of green cardamom can help fight teeth and gum infections. Therefore, eat one cardamom pod daily after every meal to prevent tooth decay. When you chew on elaichi, it increases the saliva flow that helps cleanse the teeth. It also helps control acid reflux.

4. For cough and cold, wrap one cardamom pod, a small piece of ginger, one clove and five tulsi leaves in a betel leaf and consume.

5. Boil a few black cardamom seeds in 500 ml water and reduce to half. Drink lukewarm to control vomiting.

6. To cure mouth ulcers, black cardamom seeds and mishri work well.

7. Green cardamom is an ideal solution for digestive problems as it increases the secretion of bile acid, helps prevent gastric problems, acidity and indigestion. Grind green cardamom, dry ginger and clove to make a fine powder. Ingest 1 tsp of this powder with lukewarm water whenever you have indigestion or flatulence.

8. Chew one pod of green cardamom while travelling by car, taxi or bus to keep motion sickness at bay.

9. Elaichi has diuretic properties and helps detoxify the body.

10. Use cardamom with banana leaf and amla juice to flush out kidney stones.

11. Cardamom is rich in minerals like potassium, magnesium and calcium. It is a supportive natural herb for controlling cardiovascular diseases like hypertension and regularizing heartbeat.

12. Green cardamom has an aromatic and sweet flavour. You can control bad breath by chewing cardamom seeds. Its antimicrobial effects kill oral bacteria. Therefore, chew

a pod of cardamom after every meal or whenever you need to control bad breath.

Saunf/Fennel Seeds

1. Fennel seeds are rich in dietary fibre. Therefore, they can help treat gas, cramps, indigestion, and many other digestive tract maladies. Besides being a mouth freshener, chewing saunf (2–3 gm) after every meal is good for the entire digestive system.

2. You can use fennel tea (2–3 cups daily) to control gastric problems. For making fennel tea, boil a glass of water with 1 tsp fennel seeds for 5 minutes while keeping the pot covered. Consume at lukewarm temperature.

3. Fennel seeds also contain antioxidants such as quercetin and kaempferol that help in preventing ageing and keeping skin young and fair. You can use fennel oil mixed with olive oil for a face massage to prevent wrinkles.

4. Because of fennel's alpha-pinene and creosol content, that help loosen congestion and release mucus, the seeds can help cure sinus, sore throat and bronchitis. Boil 2 tsp of these seeds with 1 tsp of liquorice powder and 1 pod of black cardamom in a glass of water.

5. Fennel seeds are useful for lactating mothers to improve milk secretion.

6. Fennel seeds help keep the body cool in summers. Use it as mouth freshener with some gulkand (sweet preserve of rose petals).

7. Soak 1 tsp fennel seeds with 1 tsp coriander seeds in a glass of water at night. Mash the ingredients and filter it the following morning. Add some mishri powder in this water and consume.

8. To prepare fennel water/ark, soak 5–6 tbsp of fennel seeds in a glass of water for 2–3 hours. Then filter the liquid and keep the water aside for later use. Make a paste of the soaked fennel seeds and soak again in the fennel water for 3 hours. Strain the water again and refrigerate the fennel water. This helps improve your appetite and reduce indigestion. Take 2–3 tbsp of fennel water mixed with half cup of water daily after lunch and dinner.

9. If you take fennel seeds with green cardamom and mishri, it will help refresh your body and brain.

10. Fennel seeds control nausea and purify blood; therefore it is good for pregnant women.

11. Fennel seeds contain vitamin C, flavonoids, amino acids and magnesium that help maintain and improve vision. Consume it with mishri in equal ratio (1 tbsp) daily at night for healthy eyesight.

12. Another formula to improve weak vision is to use fennel seeds with coriander and mishri. Grind 100 gm of fennel seeds and strain/sieve to remove wastage; keep the powder aside. Now mix coriander powder and mishri powder in equal quantity with the remaining fennel seed powder. Likewise, grind 10 gm of cardamom after removing the outer layer. Mix all the ingredients thoroughly and store in a jar. Ingest 1 tsp of this powder with lukewarm milk twice a day (morning and evening).

13. Fennel seeds can treat stomach infection like loose motion, stomach cramps, and mucus in stool. In case of infection, take 50 gm fennel seeds and roast in a pan over heat. Then mix 50 gm of plain fennel seeds in it and grind it in a mixer. Consume 2 tbsp of this powder with water three times a day.

14. Amoebiasis or amoebic dysentery: Take 20 gm fennel seeds, 20 gm coriander seeds, 20 gm cumin seeds and

20 gm dry ginger powder. Roast fennel, cumin, and coriander seeds in a pan over heat. Grind all the three to make a fine powder. Now mix all the ingredients. Consume 1 tsp of this powder three times a day with water.

15. To improve your memory, take fennel seeds with almonds and sugar candy daily.

16. Fennel seeds with coriander and mishri can control migraine. Take all three ingredients in equal quantities and grind them. Whenever you have a headache due to migraine, ingest 1 tbsp of this powder three times a day with lukewarm water.

17. Fennel seeds with harad can help you deal with loose motions.

Flaxseed/Alsi

Flax contains an essential omega-3 fatty acid, alpha-linolenic acid (ALA) that plays a crucial role within the anti-inflammatory system of our body. It contains arginine and glutamine that keep the heart healthy.

How to Start:

Whenever you begin to consume flaxseed, make sure you start with a small quantity. Firstly, grind 50 gm flaxseed (don't make fine powder) and keep it in an airtight jar in the refrigerator because ground flax spoils, or oxidizes quickly.

1. Flaxseed is extremely helpful in reducing fat due to its soluble fibre that suppresses hunger and cravings for an extended period.

2. Flaxseed contains lignans that improve metabolism.

3. Flaxseed is extremely good for regulating diastolic and systolic blood pressure because it's the richest dietary source of lignans; these nutrients act as phytoestrogens.

Phytoestrogens help reduce stress and inflammation within the arteries.

4. Flaxseed also helps alleviate hot flashes and other menopausal symptoms; it can normalize the cycle by supporting the second phase.

5. Flaxseed is the richest source of soluble fibre that helps in the digestive process.

6. Flaxseed is extremely effective in curing cough and releasing mucus naturally. If you're getting tired with a chronic cough, soak 15 gm flaxseed and 5 gm liquorice powder in a glass of water for 3–4 hours. Boil thoroughly and consume.

7. For cough, lightly roast flax in a pan. Mix some mishri and keep the powder in a jar. Take 1 tbsp of this powder with warm water for a few days; it removes mucus completely and you'll get relief from cold and cough.

8. For asthmatics, drink flaxseed tea.

9. Flaxseed oil has anti-inflammatory properties and is really good for joint pain. It contains alpha-linolenic acids that control swelling and help cure backache, nerve pain and knee pain. To control joint pain, apply flaxseed oil on your joints daily and ingest 1 tsp flaxseed oil twice daily.

10. Flaxseed is rich in phosphorus, a mineral that contributes to bone health and tissue maintenance. ALA also helps stop osteoporosis.

11. If you're experiencing burning when urinating, take 1 tsp flaxseed oil twice daily.

12. Flaxseed is good for diabetes because it reduces glucose within the blood.

13. Flaxseed oil alleviates burn wounds and helps in the healing process; apply it locally on the burn wound mixing with a little lime water 3–4 times a day.

14. It helps regulate cholesterol levels.

15. Flaxseed oil can make your skin glow. Apply flaxseed oil on your face, leave it on for 10 minutes, and wash with lukewarm water; it works as a natural cleanser. After that, rub slices of cucumber to moisturize your face. Flaxseed oil can keep wrinkles at bay.

16. Flaxseed is rich in vitamin E that is extremely beneficial for hair. The minerals and vitamins contained in flaxseed can make your hair lustrous over time.

17. Heat some flaxseed with onion juice and drop this lukewarm concoction in the affected ear (2–3 drops).

18. Flaxseed also helps reduce epileptic attacks and seizures.

Giloy/Guduchi

1. Guduchi, also known as giloy, is a powerhouse of antioxidants. It works as an immunity booster and improves the body's defence reaction.

2. Giloy may be a boon for diabetic patients because it helps lower blood glucose levels. Its alkaloids, tannins, flavonoids, saponins and cardiac glycosides are the main phytoconstituents that play an anti-diabetic role. It helps with the production of insulin and enhances the capacity to burn glucose. Make a drink that combines the juice of its stem (2 inches), a leaf of the bael plant, with a touch of turmeric daily.

3. Guduchi has mild anti-pyretic effects that can help alleviate chronic fever, especially intermittent fever. Boil a stem of giloy (4–5 inches) in a glass of water until it reduces to half the amount.

4. Make its decoction with basil leaves (4–5 leaves) and consume it with a pinch of black pepper powder.

5. You can also boil coriander seeds (1 tsp) and neem bark (1 piece) with guduchi stem (4–5 inches long) in 1 glass

of water till it becomes half and consume with a pinch of black pepper powder. You can add jaggery or honey to enhance its flavour.

6. Giloy leaves can improve blood platelets count.

7. Guduchi juice with ghee or honey also helps take care of haemoglobin levels within the body.

8. If you're asthmatic, chew a piece of giloy root for relief.

9. Giloy is extremely good for fighting digestive disorders like acidity, gastritis, loss of appetite, dyspepsia, worm infestations, etc. Regular consumption of ½ gram giloy powder with amla powder will improve digestive performance.

10. For piles, consume 20 ml guduchi juice with 100 ml A2 buttermilk.

11. 30 ml guduchi juice is extremely good for your skin. It helps purify the blood by removing toxins from the body and makes the skin flawless and glossy. Its anti-ageing properties help reduce wrinkles, dark spots, fine lines and pimples.

12. Decoction of giloy helps with all kinds of skin diseases like psoriasis, leucoderma, dermatitis, sunburn, etc. For better results, have its decoction with some A2 ghee.

13. Use of giloy with guggul is extremely common for curing ringworm.

14. Giloy is quite effective while treating gout, arthritis and even fever like chikungunya; it removes swelling and controls joint pain. Boil 1 tsp giloy root with A2 milk, add ½ tsp ginger powder and a pinch of turmeric and consume.

15. For atrophic arthritis, one should take giloy with ginger.

16. Regular consumption of giloy along with black pepper will help clear the arteries.

17. Giloy is a superb herb for mental health; its calming effect helps manage stress and anxiety. Take guduchi stem powder daily.

18. Guduchi juice is good for sexual health.

19. To improve vision, take giloy juice with amla juice daily.

20. To improve iron content, mix giloy with triphala powder and consume with pipal leaf powder and honey (twice a day).

21. Giloy leaves can also alleviate burning eyes; boil its leaves in water. Once it cools down, apply over your eyelids.

22. To cure urine infection, consume guduchi juice on an empty stomach with some honey.

23. A decoction of giloy leaves, amla and baheda works well to burn fat. Boil one glass of water with 4–5 leaves of giloy, add amla powder and baheda (half a spoon each) and some turmeric to the boiling water.

24. Giloy for liver health: Giloy protects the liver and fights against liver diseases like jaundice, hepatitis, etc. This amazing herb not only prevents scarring of liver but also stimulates the regeneration of damaged tissues. Moreover, regular consumption of its extract could be very beneficial, especially when it is taken with wheatgrass juice.

25. For feet burning sensation, mix giloy juice with neem leaves and amla and make a decoction.

26. If you're suffering from a earache, juice of giloy leaves will offer you relief.

27. The diuretic properties of guduchi act as a detox for your body. It helps purify blood and improve blood circulation; take its juice with amla juice regularly.

Harad/Chebulic Myrobalan

1. Harad, or Haritaki, is an amazing cough reliever due to its pungent, bitter, and astringent taste. Whenever you've got a cough and cold, try harad powder with honey to treat it naturally.

2. For chronic cough, use it with amla and liquorice.

3. The herb removes toxins from the body and keeps the gastrointestinal system healthy. If you take haritaki regularly, it'll help regulate weight by regulating hunger.

4. Gargle with harad water to cure a sore throat.

5. For quick relief from a migraine, grind its seeds, mix with warm water and apply on the forehead.

6. For piles or haemorrhoids, simply consume 1 tsp haritaki powder with buttermilk.

7. Haritaki water is often used as an eye wash. Soak haritaki overnight in water, preferably in an earthen pot, and use this water in the morning to scrub your eyes. Water of haritaki is found to be analgesic and anti-inflammatory; it works against conjunctivitis, as well.

8. To cure burning sensation while urinating, 2–5 gm haritaki powder with 1 tsp of honey twice a day should provide relief.

9. If you've got mouth ulcers, use harad water as a mouthwash.

10. Harad can heal wounds naturally. Simply wash the injuries with a haritaki decoction.

11. Haritaki is an excellent herb for curing all sorts of stomach problems. There are different compositions of harad mixing with other herbs that could be the answer to curing acute acidity. Harad with cumin seeds is one such combination.

Other remedies include:

a) Mix harad with black cardamom
b) Mix yellow chebulic myrobalan with black cardamom and baheda
c) Mix harad with long pepper
d) Mix chebulic myrobalan with jaggery
e) Mix harad with raisins
f) Mix haritaki with amla

12. Harad works as a natural laxative; you can use it with black cardamom and black pepper to ease constipation.

13. A composition of yellow chebulic myrobalan, baheda and mishri works well to ease out stools.

14. Good for joint pain: Try the terminalia chebula with methi. Other remedies are listed from 15–16.

15. Recipe of haritaki with dry ginger.

16. Harad with giloy—a health recipe for joint pain.

17. A pinch of harad helps reliving gastric problems in babies.

18. In case of cold and cough, rub dry ginger with yellow chebulic myrobalan in similar way and feed the child with 1 tsp honey.

19. If your child is crying at night with flatulence, rub harad on rough surface and add some jaggery.

20. Harad may be a good appetizer.

21. To cure loose motions, chew a black chebulic myrobalan like a toffee.

22. Apply harad on your teeth twice daily to keep them strong.

23. Whenever you feel a build-up of abdominal gas, take one piece of haritaki and keep it in your mouth

24. To prevent hair fall and dandruff, use haritaki oil regularly. To make oil, simply heat a cup of coconut oil in a pan with three pods of haritaki in it. Boil until brown and let it cool.

25. If you're facing acne problems, try harad powder by making a paste with boiled water.

Nutmeg/Jaiphal

1. Jaiphal contains myristicin, a compound that helps promote sleep. Moreover, it is rich in magnesium that helps scale back nerve tension. For insomnia, mix a pinch of nutmeg powder with a touch of pure ghee (preferably cow's ghee) and rub around the temples before going to sleep. It relaxes your mind and facilitates better sleep.

2. Nutmeg oil contains eugenol that helps relieve toothache naturally.

3. Nutmeg induces the secretion of varied gastric and intestinal juices that helps with the digestive process. Add a touch of nutmeg powder to your daily diet; sprinkle it on your salad or soup to improve digestion.

4. A few drops of nutmeg oil with honey can control gastritis and indigestion.

5. If you experience rheumatic pain, arthritis, gout or muscular pain, apply its oil locally. Gently massage the affected area with 3–4 drops of nutmeg oil with 1 tbsp coconut oil.

6. For a pinching pain, apply nutmeg paste directly on the aching area.

7. Nutmeg acts as a superb tonic for the brain. It contains key compounds such as myristicin and macelignan that help to ease mental stress, anxiety and depression. Myristicin also inhibits an enzyme within the brain

that contributes to Alzheimer's.

8.   Jaiphal is great for skin problems such as pimples, acne, boils, pox marks. In fact, it's utilized in some herbal and traditional medicines for enhancing skin health. Nutmeg is an essential ingredient in lotions, scrubs and cream. Jaiphal is a perfect ingredient to reinforce facial beauty. You can make natural scrubs by using powdered orange lentils and nutmeg reception. It's good for pigmentation, dark spots and freckles. Remedies listed from 9–10.

9.   Nutmeg and honey: Make a paste of a little nutmeg powder and honey and apply it on your face. Leave it for 15–20 minutes, then rinse with cold water. It'll help remove scars and brighten your skin within a few days. It also helps reduce wrinkles, signs of ageing, and other facial blemishes.

10. Nutmeg powder with cinnamon: For curing acne, make a paste with a pinch of nutmeg powder, cinnamon and honey in equal amounts and apply the mixture every morning. Keep it for around 10–15 minutes, then rinse with cold water. It helps get rid of acne and scars.

11. Being a source of potassium, jaiphal helps relax blood vessels.

12. Because of its aphrodisiac properties, nutmeg is believed to be an appropriate fix to increase male libido.

13. To control severe headaches, apply nutmeg paste (mixed with a little water) on your forehead.

14. Jaiphal for cold among kids: Nutmeg is a well-known traditional remedy for cold and cough among kids. Mix it with honey or mother's milk to cure cough and cold.

15. Add a pinch of nutmeg powder in water to reduce frequent urination.

16. Rub a pod of nutmeg on pave with some water and

apply the paste on your back.

17. Nutmeg oil for gastric problems: If you have a stomach ache, add 2–3 drops of nutmeg oil on a few black raisins and ingest.

18. Mix a pinch of nutmeg powder along with mishri (equal amount). Consume twice daily for 3–4 weeks to increase sperm count.

Lemon Juice

1. Lemon juice prevents heat stroke during the summer months.

2. Lemon juice is an age-old treatment for indigestion. Squeeze a lemon in a glass of water and add the juice of 4–5 neem leaves and a pinch of salt. It stimulates the liver into producing bile that helps food pass smoothly through the alimentary canal.

3. Lemon with 1 tsp triphala can help with any stomach problems.

4. To control loose motions and diarrhoea, 1 tbsp lemon juice with arrowroot powder and mishri will bind you up.

5. Lemon juice with honey helps to alleviate cold.

6. Lemon water contains a high amount of citrate that helps flush out kidney stones.

7. Lemon can help treat scabies or itching within two days. Boil 100 ml cold pressed coconut oil in a pan. Let it cool and add 2 tbsp lemon juice before storing it in a bottle; rub this oil on the affected area.

8. Lemon contains a flavonoid called naringenin that helps burn body fat.

9. Apply lemon directly on the scalp to get rid of dandruff.

10. Applying lemon juice with honey on the scalp directly

can prevent hair fall.

11. Lemon has anti-bacterial properties; it is also rich in vitamin C that helps treat sore throat and infection.

Multani Mitti/Fuller's Earth

Multani mitti is extremely good for skin health because it removes all impurities and dead cells. It is a traditional ingredient that can bring that elusive natural glow to your skin.

There are different methods of using this clay as facial masks:

1. Apply a smooth paste that consists of ½ cup multani mitti and 2 tbsp rose water and leave for 15 minutes.

2. Soak 2 almonds in milk overnight; grind them in the morning and blend half cup of multani mitti to form a smooth paste; add 2–3 tbsp of milk and apply this pack on your face and neck. It removes dead cells and impurities from the skin.

3. Mix 1 tsp amount of sandalwood powder and a pinch of turmeric powder in 2 tbsp of multani mitti and add 2 tbsp tomato juice to form a paste. Apply this paste on your face and wash after 10 minutes with lukewarm water. It makes your face clean and eases skin tension lines.

4. Multani mitti absorbs surplus oil and reduces the probabilities of pimples. If your skin is oily, prepare a paste that includes multani mitti (2 tbsp), sandalwood powder (1 tsp) and add a little milk. Apply this paste on your face for 20 minutes and wash off with normal water.

5. To remove dark spots from your skin, make a paste of multani mitti with mint leaf powder. Mix 1 tsp of dry

mint leaf powder and 1 tbsp of multani mitti powder with curd to form a paste and apply it on your face. Leave it to dry for 20 minutes, then wash your face with lukewarm water.

6. If you would like to lighten a suntan and pigmentation, mix some coconut oil in 2 tsp of multani mitti and apply on the affected area. Then scrub after a while and wash with normal water.

7. If your skin is rough, mix 1 tsp multani mitti, 1tsp curd, egg white/½ tsp flaxseed powder; apply this paste on your face for 20 minutes. Then wash thoroughly with lukewarm water.

8. If you've got scar marks on your skin, mix some mashed ripe papaya (1 tbsp) and honey in 2 tsp of multani mitti. Apply this paste on your face and leave it to dry; wash thoroughly with normal water.

9. If you would like wrinkle-less skin, mix 1 spoon of carrot pulp and 2 tsp of coconut oil with 2 tbsp multani mitti. Apply this paste on your face, let it dry and then wash with normal water.

10. To remove pimples, first grind some fresh neem leaves (8–10) with water; mix with 1 tbsp multani mitti to form a paste. Apply this paste on your pimples for 10 minutes, then wash with cold water.

11. Multani mitti may be mild, yet it is an effective cleanser; our ancestors used it as a shampoo. Multani mitti helps condition hair and makes it soft and silky. It also helps get rid of toxins from hair and scalp and dandruff, too.

For dry hair:

Ingredients:

- 4 tbsp multani mitti

- 1 tbsp honey
- ½ cup curd
- Half a lemon

Method:

Mix all the ingredients thoroughly; apply the paste on your scalp and hair and leave it for 20 minutes. Then wash with normal water thoroughly.

12. For greasy hair:

    Soak equal amounts of multani mitti and reetha (soap-nut) in water for 30 minutes. Then wash your head after applying this paste on your scalp and all your hair.

13. Anti-dandruff hair pack:

    Ingredients:

    - 4–5 tbsp multani mitti
    - 5–6 tbsp soaked fenugreek seeds
    - 1 tbsp lemon juice

    Method:

    Grind the soaked (overnight) fenugreek seeds to form a paste. Mix it with multani mitti and lemon juice. Now apply the paste on your scalp and hair. Leave it for 30 minutes and wash your hair with normal water.

14. A pack made of multani mitti and orange rind powder is also excellent for getting rid of dandruff. Make a paste of 4 tbsp of multani mitti powder and a couple of tbsp of orange rind powder by adding some water. Use this pack twice every week.

15. To control hair fall:

    Ingredients:

    - 4–5 tbsp multani mitti
    - 2–3 tbsp plain curd

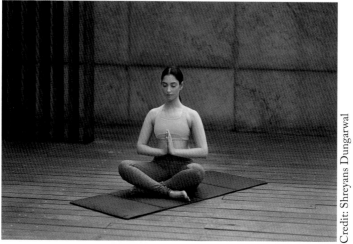

Tamannaah deep in yoga, which is a vital part of her regular workout regime.

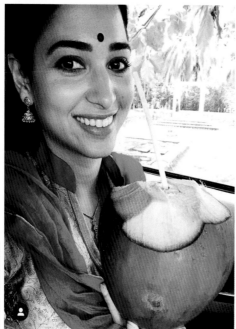

Tamannaah making sure to get healthy fats and minerals by having coconut water and its meat.

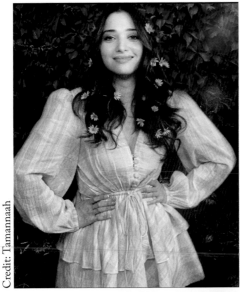

Tamannaah out in the garden, getting some fresh air.

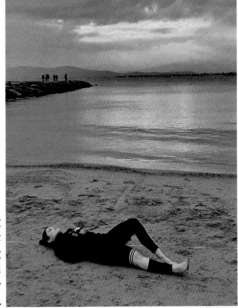

Tamannaah taking a moment to reflect on life, something we all must find time to do every now and then.

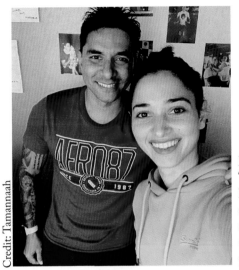

Luke helped Tamannaah get rid of her addiction to diet soda. Today, Luke has a profound influence on Tamannaah's outlook on nutrition.

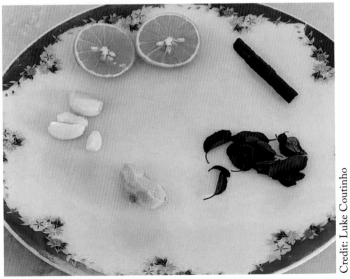

One morning in the coronavirus lockdown, Luke decided to make an immunity-boosting concoction at home. The ingredients he used were lemon juice, cinnamon, garlic, ginger and tulsi leaves.

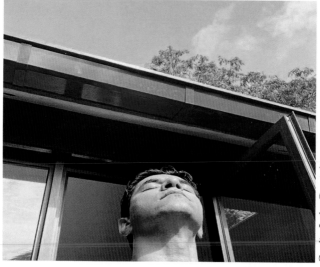

Luke taking in the sun early in the morning, readying himself for a day of discipline.

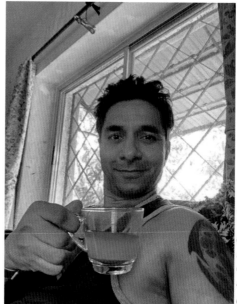

Luke enjoying his mid-morning immunity-boosting homemade tea.

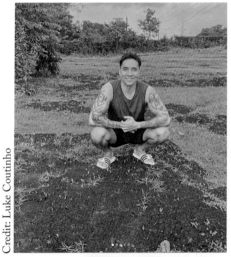

Luke out on a weekend hike, getting in some essential vitamin D and clean air.

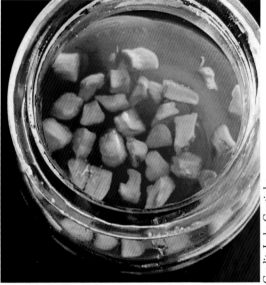

Luke also balances his immune system by having honey-infused garlic. He simply soaks chopped garlic in raw unpasteurized honey for a week and then consumes a piece each day.

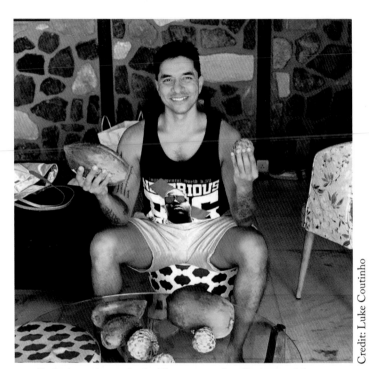

Luke beaming as he holds up some locally sourced fruits.

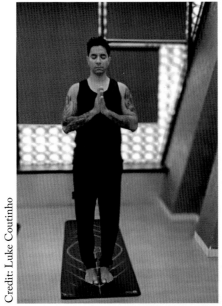

Luke initiating his
yoga routine with some
surya namaskar.

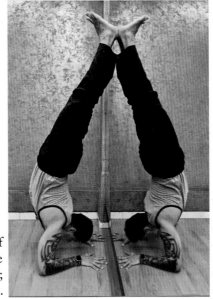

The importance of
yoga in Luke's life
cannot be overstated;
here he is in action.

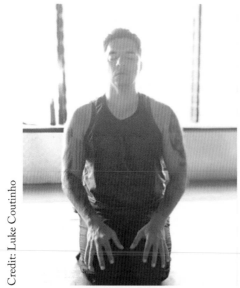

Luke
chanting 'Om'.

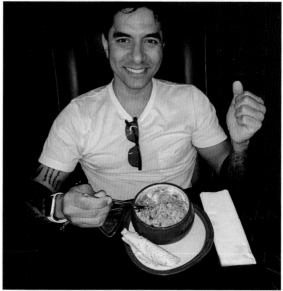

Luke enjoys his khichdi so much that he even eats it
at the movies.

- ½ tsp black pepper powder

Method:

Make a paste by mixing all the ingredients in a bowl and apply it on your hair; leave it for 20–30 minutes and then wash it off with mild shampoo.

16. For strong and healthy hair:

    To make your hair strong and healthy, mix equal quantity of reetha powder and multani mitti powder (approx. ½ cup each) and soak it in water for 30 minutes. Add 1 tsp of lemon juice to this paste and apply on your hair and scalp for 20 minutes.

17. For itchy scalp:

    Ingredients:

    - 2 tbsp multani mitti
    - 2 tbsp orange peel powder
    - 2 tbsp pomegranate peel powder
    - 2 tbsp gram flour
    - 1 cup curd

    Method:

    Mix all the ingredients in a bowl and leave it for some time. Apply it on your scalp and make sure you cover the roots well. After 20–30 minutes, wash off with normal water.

18. Multani mitti also helps enhance blood circulation.

19. Heat relief or burning sensation: multani mitti helps to scale back sunburn effects.

20. It can help plug nosebleeds; put a little piece of multani mitti near your nostrils and inhale deeply.

21. Multani mitti is a superb home remedy for heat rash. Make a paste of multani mitti powder with water and

apply over the heat rash. Let it dry for 20 minutes and wash it off with cold water.

22. Multani mitti is used as part of a cold compress for the treatment of varied problems such as muscle cramps, burns, menstrual pain, insect bites, etc.

Papaya

1. Papaya strengthens the gastrointestinal system and improves appetite. It also helps relieve constipation, indigestion and acidity. It contains papain, a proteolytic enzyme that plays a crucial role in digesting proteins faster and discouraging acid reflux. Headaches brought on by acidity and nausea can also be controlled by eating papaya daily.

2. Papaya lowers cholesterol levels because it contains powerful antioxidants like vitamin C, fibre and phytonutrients.

3. If you've got a heart problem, consume one cup of a decoction made from papaya leaves. To make decoction, boil 2–3 leaves in two cups of water till it reduces in half. Strain it and drink lukewarm.

4. Papayas are rich in potassium that plays a crucial role in reducing high blood pressure.

5. Eat a bowl of papaya daily; the fibre content will improve bowel movements and reduce the chances of piles.

6. Papaya also has anti-inflammatory properties; its unique digestive enzymes, papain and chymopapain, help scale back inflammation due to arthritis. Additionally, papaya is also rich in minerals like potassium, magnesium and copper. Its antioxidants, beta-carotene and vitamin C, can treat joint pain and bone-related health problems.

7. Papaya helps keep you full for longer durations; thus preventing frequent eating and aiding in fat loss.

8. Papayas contain antioxidants, vitamin C and vitamin E that help your skin keep radical damage at bay. Papain kills dead cells and revitalizes the skin. It also helps keep wrinkles and signs of ageing from creeping in. The healing enzymes of papaya help treat sunburn and other skin disorders.

9. Latex, another enzyme found in papaya, is beneficial while treating acne. Applying the fleshy side of a papaya on your face can cure your acne.

10. Latex also helps lighten burn scars.

11. Papaya peels can be used on your hands and face for healthy skin.

12. Papayas are rich in vitamin A and flavonoids like beta-carotene and lutein that are vital for keeping your eyes healthy.

13. Papaya acts as a superb immunity booster due to the presence of vitamin C, A, B, and K. The antioxidants present in papaya play a crucial role in improving the immunity system of the people.

14. Papain helps in easing the flow during your menstrual cycle.

15. 1 tsp juice extracted from papaya seeds is good for enlarged liver.

16. 1 tsp dried papaya seeds mixed with honey is a natural remedy for deworming.

Pippali/Long Pepper

Pippali (long pepper) is used for culinary and medicinal purposes. There are two sorts of long pepper, wet and dry. Wet long pepper is usually utilized as a cooking ingredient. Dry long pepper is usually used in powder form and has a longer shelf life.

Pippali has long been utilized in Ayurvedic treatments. It has been used to treat respiratory problems such as bronchitis, asthma, cough, infections and allergies. Additionally, pippali has been known to work against constipation, diarrhoea, stomach ache, paralysis of the tongue, cholera, chronic malaria, viral fever, diseases of the spleen, gonorrhoea and tumours.

1. Long pepper cures cough and cold by removing extra mucus.

   • Pippali with dry ginger

   Ingredients:

   • 0.5 gm long pepper powder
   • ¼ tsp dry ginger powder
   • ¼ tsp turmeric powder

   Method:

   Mix all the ingredients in ¼ cup of water and add 1 tsp of honey.

   • Pippali with black pepper

   Ingredients:

   • 10 gm piper longum root
   • 5 gm long pepper
   • 10 gm black pepper
   • 10 gm dry ginger

   Method:

   Grind the ingredients well to form a fine powder and keep in an airtight jar. Ingest 2 gm of this powder with honey twice daily to cure a cold.

- Roast long pepper in A2 ghee and consume ¼ tsp.
- Consume 1 gm pippali powder with honey.
- Boil 3 gm long pepper powder in a cup of water and add some jaggery. Now, you can sip it like tea.
- Pippali with baheda for chronic cough:

Ingredients:

- 10 gm piper longum root
- 5 gm long pepper
- 10 gm baheda
- 10 gm dry ginger

Method:

Grind all the ingredients to form a fine powder and keep it in a jar. Now ingest 3 gm regularly.

2. Pippali effectively treats different respiratory disorders like asthma, bronchitis, sinus, allergic congestion, etc. You'll get relief from asthma by consuming 1 gm pippali powder daily with honey.

3. Pippali with dry ginger for asthma:

Ingredients:

- 10 gm long pepper
- 10 gm black pepper
- 10 gm dry ginger

Method:

Grind them to form a fine powder. Now, ingest 2 gm of this powder with honey 2–3 times a day

4. Boil 2 gm of long pepper powder in 4 cups of water till it reduces to half. This pippali decoction can alleviate asthmatic issues.

5. For treating other respiratory problems like sinus, bronchitis, allergies, ingest 0.5 gm of pippali powder with honey or jaggery twice daily.

6. Piper longum has piperine which helps fight certain parasites known to damage the gastrointestinal system. Piperine defends it by forming a liner in the intestines. Besides digestion, it also helps improve appetite and treat heartburn, intestinal gas, stomach ache and diarrhoea.

7. For indigestion, use pippali powder with dry ginger and ajwain.

8. Piper longum is extremely good for those who suffer from gas formation and abdominal pain.

9. Pippali with harad is a good traditional hack for acid reflux.

10. Pippali acts as a sedative for those suffering from insomnia. Consume 3–5 gm of pipramul powder with double the amount of jaggery.

11. Long pepper has anti-inflammatory properties. Simply, take pippali (0.5–1 gm in a day) with honey. Prepare the paste of pippali (with water) and apply on the affected area.

12. Long pepper is an age old folk medicine for headaches because of its anti-bacterial properties. Make a paste of long pepper root powder with water and apply on the forehead.

13. You can ingest pippali powder (3 gm) with warm water to relieve a migraine.

14. Blend and boil 1 gm long pepper powder, 5–7 basil leaves, ½ tsp turmeric powder, 5 gm crushed ginger; this mix will help alleviate fever.

15. Pippali is good for those suffering from hemiplegia. Take 1 gm of pippali powder with 2–3 gm of ghee twice daily.

16. For sciatica pain, boil pippali in water, add 1 tsp A2 ghee and consume.

17. For controlling hiccups, 1 gm long pepper powder with honey or water.

18. For vomiting, you can have pippali with liquorice.

    Ingredients:
    - 10 gm long pepper
    - 10 gm liquorice (mulethi)
    - 20 gm rock sugar (mishri)
    - 1 lemon wedge

    Method:

    Mix all the ingredients in a glass of water and add a few drops of juice.

19. Take equal amounts of pippali, rock salt, turmeric powder and mustard oil. Mix all well and make a paste. Now apply this paste on the affected tooth to cure toothache.

20. Grind 10 gm each of these ingredients: pippali dry ginger, rock salt and mace; add 1 tbsp honey. Add a little of this mix on your palm with a little honey to form a paste and rub on your gums.

21. Grind equal amounts of piper longum root with green cardamom and store in a jar. Ingest 3 gm of this powder mixing it with A2 ghee to improve heart health.

22. For heartburn, ingest 1 gm pippali powder with 1 tsp honey twice a day; it also helps cure heart conditions.

23. For constipation, take 1 gm pippali powder and 1 gm harad powder. Add 1 tsp of honey and ingest.

24. For curing haemorrhoids, consume 1 gm pippali powder and a pinch of turmeric with ½ cup fresh yoghurt daily, in the morning (after breakfast) and night (after dinner).

25. For blood in urine, take ¼ tsp pippali powder with ½ tsp roasted cumin seeds powder and blend.

26. To cure blood in stool, pippali with bitter apple root, in equal quantities, works well.

27. For treating menstrual cramps, take 2 tbsp fresh carrot juice and 0.5 gm pippali powder with ½ cup warm water.

28. For improving low libido (men), take 0.5 gm pippali with ½ tsp ashwagandha powder and 1 tsp ghee and consume with ¼ cup water.

29. Use 0.5 gm pippali, ½ tsp asparagus and 1 tsp ghee and consume with ¼ cup water for improving low libido (women).

30. Pippali and its root are given to mothers after delivery to ensure the uterus retains its normal size.

31. Long pepper can control stomach cramps. Take harad and pippali (1 gm each) and consume with warm water twice daily.

32. Long pepper has components that are known to protect the liver. Boil one crushed long pepper with one glass of warm water and consume by adding ¼ tsp ajwain powder.

33. For liver and spleen enlargement, make a decoction of 1 gm pippali and 5 gm pipramul. Boil both the powders with one glass of water. Strain and drink.

34. To reduce excess fat, use 2 gm pippali with 5 gm honey, three times daily.

35. If you've got arthritis, knee pain or any joint pain, collect some roots of old long pepper plant and dry them in the sun. Grind these roots to form a fine powder and keep in a jar. Ingest 3–5 gm of this powder with warm milk or water to cure any sort of joint or body ache. This is often a superb remedy that provides relief within a few hours.

36. For muscle pain, mix both bitter apple root and long pepper root powder in equal amounts. Have 1 tsp of this powder with a glass of warm water in the morning.

37. Whenever you've got any sort of skin issue, prepare a paste of pippali powder with water and apply on the affected area (twice daily).

38. For skin rashes, mix 0.5 gm long pepper powder, 2 tbsp aloe vera juice, ¼ tsp turmeric powder with water and consume on an empty stomach.

39. Piper longum root has anti-diabetic and anti-hyperlipidaemic properties.

40. To cure loose motions, take ¼ tsp of pippali powder with a glass of buttermilk twice daily.

Pumpkin Seeds

1. Pumpkin seeds are a rich source of zinc, selenium and magnesium. Low levels of selenium can lead to an enlarged prostate while zinc enables testosterone. Consume 1 tsp raw or sprouted seeds to improve male reproductive health.

2. The high zinc level in pumpkin seeds helps enhance immunity, heal wounds and support normal growth.

3. Pumpkin seed nutrients help to increase good cholesterol (HDL). Moreover, its high level of antioxidants, zinc, magnesium and essential fatty acids support your heart health. Therefore, eat a few seeds as a snack or an ingredient in a main dish.

4. Seeds of pumpkin not only improve sleep, but also help treat depression. They contain niacin which helps in the production of the neurotransmitter serotonin that helps regulate moods and helps the production of melatonin.

5. Pumpkin seeds have been used for their anthelmintic (antiworm) properties since ancient times. It is believed

that a cucurbitacin present in these seeds paralyses the intestinal worms and helps to expel worms from the intestine.

6. Pumpkin seeds are rich in antioxidants. They are also an excellent source of magnesium that plays an important role in bone formation.

7. Pumpkin seed oil has phytoestrogens (plant-based oestrogens) that mimic the oestrogen (female sex hormone) and reduce post-menopausal symptoms.

8. Pumpkin seed oil is rich in zinc that helps reduce post-menopausal symptoms like hot flashes, headaches, vaginal dryness, joint pain and insomnia.

9. Pumpkin seeds are a rich source of zinc, vitamin A, vitamin E, beta-carotene, lutein and zeaxanthin that protects the eyes and aids proper vision. Zinc facilitates vitamin A in travelling from the liver to the retina which sequentially creates melanin (pigment that protects and imparts colour to the eye).

10. Pumpkin seeds have a good ratio of omega-6 and omega-3, hence lowering LDL cholesterol. Phytosterols present in these seeds are potent in the reduction of bad cholesterol. In addition to that, phytosterols help reduce the absorption of bad cholesterol (LDL) from your diet.

11. Pumpkin seeds are a nutritional powerhouse. They are a good source of plant-based proteins that work as building blocks for the human body.

12. Antioxidants like carotenoids and vitamin E help reduce free radicals, provide moisture to the skin and keep you young.

13. Magnesium in pumpkin seeds regulates normal muscle and nerve function.

14. Folate present in pumpkin seeds is a precursor of

genetic material (DNA) and other essential amino acids. Hence, it is beneficial for pregnant women.

15. Women after childbirth have weak pelvic floor muscles and often complain of passing urine (in small amounts) during exercise, while sneezing or suddenly getting up from a seated position. Pumpkin seeds help strengthen pelvic floor muscles.

16. Pumpkin seeds help increase nitric oxide that leads to better regulation of blood pressure.

17. Pumpkin seeds are a good source of iron that helps eliminate symptoms of anaemia like fatigue, dark skin, etc.

18. Pumpkin seeds are rich in zinc, magnesium, iron and copper that are important for brain function.

Raisin/Munakka

1. Munakka helps control vertigo.

2. Grind 8–10 raisins, 10 gm liquorice and 10 gm mishri into a fine powder. Using this mixture like snuff is known to be very effective against headaches brought on acidity.

3. Raisins are good for curing any type of oral problem including mouth ulcers. Boil 8–10 raisins and 3–4 leaves of blackberry in a glass of water for 10 minutes. Gargle with this decoction (lukewarm) 3–4 times a day.

4. To control nose bleeds, put 3–4 drops of grapes or raisin juice in the nostrils. Even a whiff of this juice will provide immediate relief.

5. Munakka has anti-bacterial properties and works well to control bad breath due to cough or indigestion. It helps release mucus and improves digestion. If you eat 5–10 raisins daily, you can get rid of bad breath without a mouth freshener.

6. To cure a chest wound, eat munakka with paddy seeds. All you need is 10 gm paddy seeds, 10 gm raisins and 100 ml water. Soak the paddy seeds and raisins in water overnight. Then mash them thoroughly with your fingers to make a paste. Ingest 6 gm of this paste with honey 3–4 times in a day.

7. To control vomiting, use the remedy mentioned in point 6.

8. For chronic or dry cough, grind the following and consume 1 tsp of it on an empty stomach: 10 gm raisin, 10 gm piper longum, 10 gm black pepper and 10 gm dates.

9. Boil 10–20 raisins in a glass of A2 milk for ten minutes and drink it at night as a laxative and to cure constipation.

10. Roasted raisins with a pinch of rock salt at night before going to sleep can be very effective against piles.

11. A decoction of raisin, figs, fennel seeds, rose leaves and amla is very effective and safe.

12. Munakka with cumin seeds and black pepper works well to cure constipation naturally.

13. Raisins with fennel seeds cure acidity. Soak 10 gm raisins and 5 gm fennel seeds in 100 ml water at night and mash them in the morning. Drink this water on an empty stomach after sieving.

14. Raisins are a rich source of iron and vitamin B complex. By eating 5–10 raisins daily, you can increase your haemoglobin level and keep anaemia at bay.

15. In order to cure a bedwetting disorder, take two raisins, remove the seeds and add black pepper seeds in a 1:1 proportion. Give it to your child before going to sleep at night regularly for 2–3 weeks.

16. Raisins are full of nutrients and work as a complete health tonic. They help make your body healthy and

energetic. Therefore, eat 5–10 raisins daily, soaking in water overnight.

17. Munakka is a good source of polyphenols, a phytonutrient that is good for the eyes. Its antioxidants and other nutrients are good for ocular health and protect our eyes from glaucoma, night blindness, cataract, etc.

18. Raisins are a rich source of calcium and the micronutrient boron that help to strengthen our bones and teeth. Include it in your daily diet and ingest 5–10 raisins daily.

19. Raisins are extremely helpful in gaining weight due to its iron and natural sugars, sucrose and glucose. Roast raisins (7–10) in A2 ghee.

20. Raisins have certain photochemicals that are necessary for dental health. By eating 5–7 raisins daily, you'll protect your teeth from cavities and other gum problems.

21. Raisins contain potassium that helps reduce tension in blood vessels.

22. To reduce high fever, soak 25 raisins in 200 ml of water for a few hours. Then, mash the raisins into the water and add half a lemon's juice. Now, strain the water into a cup and ingest twice a day.

23. Soak 10 raisins and 1 fig in half a cup of water for a few hours. At night, remove the soaked raisins and fig from the water and boil with a glass of milk.

24. Make a healthy paste of 20 gm raisins, 20 gm piper longum, 20 gm dates, 20 gm honey and 20 gm A2 ghee. Grind thoroughly to make a paste and consume 5 gm daily.

Sabja/Sweet Basil Seeds

1. Sweet basil seeds are exceptionally high in fibre. These fibre-rich seeds have a higher level of mucilage

(soluble fibre), thus helping regulate bowel movements and improving digestion.

2. Sabja seeds expand up to 30 times their original volume when soaked. The gelatinous mass of those seeds will keep you full for a longer time. Sweet basil seeds contain high levels of protein; about 14 per cent of its content is slow to digest and keeps you full. Add these seeds to your smoothie, falooda, shake or water.

3. Sweet basil seeds are one of the richest sources of omega-3 fatty acids. Higher level of omega-3 helps reduce cholesterol.

4. The antioxidants present in sweet basil seeds reduce the assembly of free radicals within the body and reduce the effects of degenerative diseases like Alzheimer's.

5. Sweet basil seeds help maintain blood glucose level by slowing down the release of sugars. They also help increase secretion of insulin in Type II diabetes, thus maintaining blood glucose level.

6. Sabja seeds are rich in antioxidants and even have cholesterol and triglyceride-lowering properties. These properties help scale back free radicals from the body and reduce chances of cardiovascular complications.

7. Sweet basil seeds are known to possess anti-bacterial, anti-fungal and antiviral properties. They assist in the fight against a wide spectrum of pathogens and keep you healthy.

8. The cooling properties of sabja seeds also help reduce acidity. They protect the layer around the stomach and reduce the production of acid.

9. Sweet basil seeds have anti-anxiety and anti-depressant properties that help you stay in a good mood.

10. Sweet basil seeds are rich in antioxidants and thus make your skin more radiant. Apply powdered seeds mixed

with cold pressed coconut oil for about 20 minutes and rinse; this may make your skin soft and supple; it also reduces blemishes.

11. Sabja seeds also help fight skin diseases like eczema and psoriasis. Simply apply a paste of pre-soaked (about 20 minutes) seeds along with turmeric powder on the affected skin area.

12. Sabja seeds are rich in vitamin K, protein and minerals like iron that help make your hair stronger and more radiant.

13. Sweet basil seeds are very commonly referred to as falooda seeds due to their cooling properties. You can make a falooda with sabja or add it to milkshake and lemonade, or simply add these seeds to a bottle of water while going out; it'll protect you from the scorching heat of the sun.

14. Sweet basil seeds also help treat bad breath, gum diseases and mouth ulcers. Sabja seeds help fight against streptococcus mutans, the pathogen that causes oral cavities. Herbal mouthwash can be prepared by using sweet basil seed oil.

15. Sweet basil seeds are rich in vitamin A and beta-carotene. Vitamin A acts as an antioxidant booster for the retina and also helps arrest loss of vision (macular degeneration) and development of cataract.

16. The carminative effect of basil seeds cures all general stomach-associated ailments like acidity, flatulence, constipation and irregular movement. Mucilage (soluble fibre), the main content of soaked sabja seeds, helps relieve constipation. They ease movement and protect the interior lining of the intestine.

17. Basil seeds are very useful for curing a bladder infection. The antibacterial properties of basil seeds help us fight infection. Actually, the most common reason for urinary

infection is a smaller amount of water intake and sabja seeds help us to improve our water intake. Consume 1 tbsp soaked sabja seeds for best results.

18. Sabja seeds are rich in antioxidants and flavonoids like vicenin and oreton; they act as an immunity booster. The rich properties of basil seeds help us fight general infections like cold and cough. Due to its anti-inflammatory properties, sweet basil seeds also help alleviate muscle pain brought on by excessive coughing.

19. An aminoalkanoic acid, L-tryptophan, that isn't formed by our body, is present in basil seeds. L-tryptophan helps with the release of the hormones serotonin and melatonin. These hormones are referred to as natural sleep inducers.

Moringa/Horseradish Tree/Drumstick/Sehjan

The health benefits of moringa or sehjan are:

1. Moringa has been promoted by the World Health Organization (WHO) as an alternative to imported food sources to treat malnutrition.

2. Research says that the dry leaves of moringa contain nine times more protein than yoghurt, ten times more vitamin A than carrot, twenty-five times more iron than spinach, fifteen times more potassium than bananas, seventeen times more calcium than milk, and seven times more vitamin C than an orange.

3. Moringa leaves are rich in minerals like calcium, potassium, zinc, magnesium, iron and copper.

4. Vitamins like beta-carotene of vitamin A, vitamin B such as choline, folic acid, pyridoxine and nicotinic acid, vitamin C, D and E are also present in moringa.

5. Moringa contains phytochemicals like sterols, tannins, terpenoids, saponins, alkaloids, phenolics and flavonoids like isoquercitin, isothiocyanates, quercetin, kaemfericitin, and glycoside compounds. Various amino acids like histamine, arginine, tryptophan, lysine, threonine, phenylalanine, leucine, isoleucine, methionine, and valine are also found in moringa. Its leaves contain an array of amino acids, making it particularly beneficial for vegans and vegetarians to obtain a sufficient protein supply.

6. Moringa leaves treat hyperglycaemia, asthma, flu, heartburn, dyslipidaemia, malaria, syphilis, diarrhoea, pneumonia, scurvy, headaches, bronchitis, skin diseases, and eye and ear infections. It also reduces blood pressure and cholesterol and acts as an anti-cancer, antioxidant, antimicrobial, anti-atherosclerotic, anti-diabetic agent, and a neuroprotectant.

7. Moringa has also been observed to be an effective treatment against a wide array of liver diseases, such as both chronic and acute hepatitis, cirrhosis of the liver, fatty degeneration of the liver, and metabolic liver disease brought about by alcohol and drug abuse. This is because moringa not only halts toxicity; it also helps reverse the causes of these diseases.

8. It helps lower blood sugar levels. The effect maybe induced by glucoside and fibre that are present in moringa leaf powder.

9. Moringa powder is rich in vitamin A and zinc that encourages hair growth and keeps it in good condition. In addition, moringa powder is rich in vitamins B, C and E, biotin, and inositol that provide nutrients to help improve scalp circulation and maintain capillaries that carry blood to the follicles.

10. Moringa might work as a galactagogue, an agent that induces milk secretion. A single serving of moringa

contains about 3 times the iron of spinach. Iron is essential to enriching the blood, carrying life, energy and oxygen to our muscles and organs.

11. Moringa fights against fatigue by providing iron and vitamin A to the human body. Iron is very useful for the prevention of fatigue in our body.

12. Moringa helps maintain healthy skin and prevent ageing as it is rich in vitamin A and vitamin E. Vitamin A is necessary for healthy, radiant skin and vitamin E protects cells from oxidative stress helping to fight the signs of ageing. Antioxidants are essential for protecting, repairing and preventing cell damage, minimizing the ageing process. They help counteract oxidative stress and the effects of free radicals. Free radicals are unstable molecules that damage collagen, causing skin dryness, fine lines, wrinkles and premature ageing.

13. Moringa also contains cytokines and zeatin which are known to delay ageing in humans.

14. Moringa benefits have super immune-boosting powers that help body cells stay strong and fight germs. Moringa leaves are full of iron and vitamin A, and in this case, both are essential for the normal function of the immune system.

15. Oleifera is a powerful and natural adaptogen that not only helps the body cope with stress but can enhance general health and performance.

16. Moringa is a great source of vitamin A that helps maintain visual function.

17. Moringa leaves are a rich source of vitamin K, protein and calcium, all of which support bone health.

18. It also contains the amino-acid tryptophan that improves neurotransmitter function. Tryptophan is

sought out by many as it's the neurotransmitter that secretes serotonin, our happiness hormone.

19. Moringa leaves help alleviate symptoms of anxiety, vertigo and vomiting.

20. Moringa may be a good source of calcium that helps keep bones and teeth healthy. Just add a few drumsticks to dal or sambhar daily. Alternatively, dry its leaves, make a powder and consume ½ tsp with milk, curd or salad.

21. Moringa helps in the purification of blood which treats many skin problems, so add drumsticks to your daily diet and make your skin beautiful.

How to use moringa for glowing skin:

22. Make a paste of sehjan leaves and apply on the face. After 15–20 minutes, wash your face with lukewarm water. This will make your skin glow, keep it pimple-free, and delay ageing.

23. Extract the juice of 3–4 drumsticks by grinding and straining; then squeeze a lemon into the mix. It will rejuvenate your skin and make it shine.

24. Moringa oil is a rich source of behenic acid that forms a protective barrier against the skin and provides moisture. Moringa oil also helps obviate pimple marks and blemishes. Therefore, massage your face with a few drops of moringa oil every day for a clear complexion.

25. Sehjan has this very amazing property of water purification. In the past, drumstick leaves powder and seeds were mixed with water to remove its impurities. The water was then strained and consumed.

26. Sehjan helps strengthen the gastrointestinal system. Drumsticks are rich in fibre that helps manage bowel movement and treats constipation. It's also good to treat

other stomach-related problems like loose motions, dysentery, cholera, diarrhoea and jaundice.

27. Grind equal quantities of moringa root, mustard and ginger and prepare tablets of 1 gm each. Consume 1 tablet every morning and evening. It cures spleen issues and improves digestive power.

28. Mix 9 gm sehjan root juice and 1 gm ginger juice; consume every morning and evening to enhance digestive power.

29. For blocked nose and congestion, simply boil 5–6 moringa seed pods in 2 litres of water. Inhale the steam from this water twice daily.

30. In Ayurveda, sehjan is an age-old treatment for migraines. Take 15–20 washed drumstick leaves and make a paste. Apply the paste to your forehead and other affected areas of your head. Now, lie down comfortably, close your eyes and rest for about 20 minutes.

31. Rub the dry seeds of moringa on a rough stone and inhale. The scent helps alleviate headaches.

32. Drumstick root and jaggery are quite effective in curing headache. Mix equal quantities of juice from its root and jaggery; use 1 drop of this mixture during an Ayurvedic nasal massage.

33. Zinc present in drumstick helps increase sperm count and improve semen viscosity. Therefore, it is also referred to as Indian Viagra. Consume moringa for better sexual health.

34. At first, boil a few pieces of drumstick bark in about ½ litre water for 5 minutes or so. Add 1 tsp of honey and consume. Drink this decoction regularly to obviate premature ejaculation.

35. Boil 7–10 moringa flowers with 200 ml of milk for 2–4 minutes and drink while it's warm, twice daily

(morning and evening). This will help improve your sexual health.

36. Sehjan leaf juice or powder helps get rid of stomach worms in kids and adults.

37. Sehjan has analgesic properties and helps scale back muscular pain, stomach ache, rib pain, among other aches. It also reduces swelling and inflammation. Use sehjan bark to scale back internal swelling and inflammation. Simply, make a paste of sehjan tree bark by grinding with the help of water and apply on the affected area.

38. Consume 1 tsp of drumstick powder with water on an empty stomach to cure constipation.

39. Sehjan may be a rich source of vitamin B complex and also treats stomach-related general problems like indigestion. To cure mouth and throat ulcers, boil 1 tsp moringa root in 300 ml water until it is reduced to one-fourth of its original quantity. Gargle with this decoction 2–3 times a day

40. Moringa is known for its antibacterial properties and research has shown that moringa bark decoction helps treat UTIs. Drinking moringa leaf tea has a diuretic action that also helps fight bacterial infection.

41. In Ayurveda, drumstick is understood for its properties as a *rakt shodhak* (blood purifier) and *yakrit shodhana* (liver cleanser).

42. If you're suffering from a earache, a few drops of sehjan leaf juice in the ear canal will help. Repeat the method after 4 hours if pain persists.

43. Moringa's antibacterial properties help reduce the chances of wound infection. Apply a paste of its leaves on the wounded area and cover with cotton. Wash after a few hours.

44. Sehjan could be a potential medicine that helps regulate flatulence and stomach ache with other ingredients. 100 gm drumstick bark, 15 gm dry ginger and 4 gm asafoetida; grind all and consume ½ tsp every day.

45. Bronchial asthma is triggered by allergies that results in contraction of bronchioles and difficulty in breathing. Sehjan seeds have the potential to treat asthma. Having 3 gm moringa seeds powder with water helps scale back symptoms of asthma. Additionally, it improves the respiratory function of the lungs.

46. For bronchitis, mix drumstick root juice with ginger juice (equal quantity). Consume 1 tbsp of this mixture every morning and evening.

47. Grind a few drumstick leaves and make a paste. Apply this paste on the eyelids and tie with a strip of fabric. Let it stay for about an hour and wash gently. Repeat the method twice daily to treat conjunctivitis.

48. For corneal opacity, simply grind sufficient drumstick leaves and extract 50 ml juice. Mix this juice with 1 tbsp of honey and apply as eyeliner. Let it stay for a few hours and repeat the process twice daily.

49. Mix drumstick leaf juice and honey in equal quantities and put one drop on each eye to reduce swelling and pain. Repeat the process for a few days for better results. Store the mixture in a refrigerator.

50. Sehjan has a high amount of calcium and other minerals like zinc, magnesium and potassium. Calcium is the building block of bones and teeth while magnesium helps with the overall functioning of the body.

Tulsi/Holy Basil

1. Pyorrhoea: Brush your teeth with tulsi leaf powder.
2. Tulsi juice is a natural deworming shot.

3. Lumbar backache: Regular consumption of tulsi leaves helps reduce lower back pain. Prepare a decoction of tulsi with ginger and black cardamom and drink/use regularly.

4. Diabetes: Regular consumption of holy basil leaves can aid in balancing various bodily processes. It counters elevated blood sugar levels and can help in keeping diabetes under control. For diabetics, try powder of dry basil leaves with neem and bael leaves; it shows good results in most diabetic cases.

5. Influenza or flu: Basil tea with ginger and clove works effectively in case of influenza or flu; its antibiotic, anti-viral and anti-bacterial properties help to regulate fever. For basil tea: Boil 1 cup of water in a pan with some crushed ginger. Add 7–9 tulsi leaves, 3–4 crushed black pepper pods and 1 clove. Bring to a boil, strain and drink.

6. A decoction of tulsi with cardamom can regulate fever. Simply boil 12–15 fresh leaves with cardamom powder in 500 ml water until it reduces in half. Then drink it warm with honey.

7. For high forehead temperature, prepare a paste of dry basil and place cold strips on the forehead.

8. Tulsi ark (holy basil water) can also help control high fever. 1 tsp of tulsi ark can reduce high fever along with cold water strips.

9. A decoction that consists of basil leaves, ginger and black pepper is an ancient remedy for cold and cough. The tulsi plant's mucus-releasing properties make this decoction a good remedy for alleviating cough and cold in children, as well.

10. For ailments like sinus, rub tulsi juice on nose, ear and forehead of the child daily right before bedtime.

11. Eating basil leaves (7–9) daily provides relief from acidity.

12. For curing stomach ache, take 20–22 leaves of basil and grind to form a thick paste. Apply this paste in and around the naval area.

13. Tulsi for burning eyes: Burning eyes may be a common problem that usually occurs due to continuous use of computer or electronic devices. Tulsi ark cures this burning easily.

14. Joint pain and muscular pain: Tulsi contains powerful enzyme-inhibiting oils that lower inflammation. This can help alleviate joint pain. Certain studies have shown that basil contains high quantities of beta-caryophyllene that is beneficial for arthritis. Consume its leaves to improve the condition.

15. Tulsi stem with honey helps to strengthen joints.

16. Take equal amounts of basil roots, stems, leaves and seeds and dry thoroughly in sunlight. Grind into a powder and store in an airtight jar. Use 1 tsp of this powder with old jaggery daily. It controls inflammation due to arthritis, gout and joint pain.

17. If you've got nerve or muscle pain, use basil juice or its decoction. Simply boil 12–15 basil leaves in one cup of water, reduce to half, and drink it twice or three times a day.

18. Make oil of basil and apply on the affected area to cure pain. To prepare basil oil, boil 20–25 leaves in 100 gm of mustard oil thoroughly and strain. Massage the affected area with this oil twice daily or when required.

19. Mouth ulcers are bound to reduce if you chew 4–5 basil leaves daily for a week.

20. Tulsi is good for the liver and is utilized to treat conditions like hepatitis. Eat 10–12 washed tulsi leaves daily in the morning.

21. Basil leaves can cure skin disorders, whether consumed or applied topically. For skin disease, apply tulsi ark or rub fresh leaves on the affected area.

22. Basil juice for earache: In case of ear pain, boil 10–12 tulsi leaves in some mustard oil with garlic juice. Let it cool and strain the oil into a jar. Pour 2–3 drops in the ear canal to alleviate pain.

23. Dizziness or vertigo: Take 1 tsp of basil leaves juice along with 1 tsp of honey. To extract basil juice, simply crush 12–15 leaves and press through a sieve.

24. Piles: Basil seeds help control blood in piles.

25. A decoction of basil leaves, ginger and black pepper works as an excellent natural medicine to reduce swelling of throat glands.

26. Pharyngitis can be treated with a decoction of basil leaves and black pepper.

27. Tulsi is a superb remedy for respiratory health problems such as bronchitis, asthma, cold and cough, etc. Use its leaves along with ginger and honey. Simply crush some ginger and extract 1 tsp of its juice. Now mix 1 teaspoon honey and ingest immediately. This home remedy can also be used for children but the dosage will be half.

28. Basil helps regulate acid levels, thus eliminating the risk of developing kidney stones. It also helps getting rid of kidney stones. To remove urinary calculi, consume 1 tsp of tulsi ark with honey daily.

29. Chew 12 leaves of basil twice daily to prevent stress.

Triphala

Triphala is a recognized and highly effective polyherbal Ayurvedic medicine. It consists of the fruits of three plant species—amla (emblica officinalis), bahera (terminalia bellerica), andharitaki (terminalia chebula)—and may be a cornerstone of gastrointestinal and rejuvenatory treatment. The major constituents of the formula are tannins, gallic acid, ellagic acid and chebulinic acid, all potent antioxidants that may account, at least in part, for the immunomodulatory activity. Triphala also contains other bioactive compounds such as flavonoids (e.g., quercetin and luteolin), saponins, anthraquinones, amino acids, fatty acids and various carbohydrates. The polyphenols in triphala modulate the human gut microbiome and thereby promote the growth of beneficial bifidobacteria and lactobacillus while inhibiting the growth of undesirable gut microbes. The bioactivity of triphala is elicited by gut microbiota to generate a variety of anti-inflammatory compounds.

Research has found triphala to be potentially effective for several clinical uses such as:

1. Laxative

2. Appetite stimulation

3. Reduction of hyperacidity

4. Antioxidant and free radical scavenging

5. Anti-inflammatory

6. Immunomodulating

7. Hypoglycaemia

8. Prevention of dental caries

9. Antipyretic, analgesic, antibacterial, antineoplastic, antimutagenic

10. Wound healing

11. Anti-stress

12. Adaptogenic

13. Anti-cancer

14. Hepatoprotective

15. Chemoprotective and radioprotective effects
16. Promoting proper digestion and absorption of food
17. Reducing of serum cholesterol levels
18. Improving circulation
19. Relaxing bile ducts
20. Maintaining homeostasis of the endocrine

Hacks for Healthy Living

Gut-Friendly Foods

There are a lot of myths around fermented foods like dosas, idlis, dhoklas; whether they are good or bad for you. A lot of people complain about bloating and flatulence, indigestion and acidity, after eating fermented foods.

Fermented foods are extremely healthy for you. If you suffer from indigestion, acidity, bloating and flatulence, you can't blame your food or your staple diet. You need to work on strengthening your digestive system and making lifestyle changes. In grains and beans, phytic acid produces most of the bloating and indigestion. During the fermentation process, phytic acid is broken down and that's why you're able to digest the food better without any gas or acidity. It's a good idea to ferment and break down phytic acid, because it blocks the absorption of minerals from the food that you eat. The breaking down of phytic acid actually allows for the bioavailability and absorption of vitamins and minerals, and then onwards to your billions of cells.

Fermentation also gives rise to lactobacilli that produce an array of vitamins, especially of the B variety, including the synthesis of vitamin B12, a common deficiency. Lactobacilli also give rise to folic acid, riboflavin, niacin, thymidine, even vitamin K, vitamin B12 and certain antibiotic and anti-carcinogenic properties.

Fermented food also lasts longer and helps develop healthy gut bacteria in your intestines. Almost everyone has an incorrect ratio of good and bad bacteria; that is why we have indigestion, bloating, acidity, flatulence, IBS, leaky gut syndrome and malnourishment because most of the minerals and vitamins from the food that we eat don't get absorbed in our body. When you have the correct ratio of good and bad bacteria, you have proper assimilation of food, proper digestion, good bowel movement and good colon health. All of which you receive from fermented food.

Of course, you need to beware of roadside fermented food covered in reused butter and oil. Stick to homemade dosas, idlis or dhoklas or any fermented food item. The problem is never with your staple foods. It is with your lifestyle. So go enjoy all the fermented foods!

Benefits of Keeping the Body Alkaline

Alkaline food boosts our energy dramatically. Oxygen breeds in an alkaline medium. All the tissues, cells, body fluids are in their active state and function smoothly in the presence of oxygen. The output is better energy levels! An alkaline diet also helps us get a better night's sleep and one that is infinitely more restful, helping us to keep our energy levels high throughout a busy day.

Alkaline food keeps our body functioning at its optimal level. All the metabolic processes, including digestion in the gut run smoothly in an alkaline body pH. Stomach digestion is an exception here, as it needs an acidic pH.

Prevents diseases: Several research studies have shown that a diet low in acid-producing food and rich in alkaline-forming food keeps bones and muscles strong, improves heart health and brain function, reduces arthritis, prevents kidney stones, and lowers the risk of type 2 diabetes. Alkaline food is also known to slow down the ageing process. Free radicals accelerate the ageing process. An acidic environment is conducive to free radical production, whereas an alkaline environment coupled with antioxidants helps reduce or neutralize the free radicals, which in a way, slows down the ageing process.

Cancer cells flourish in an acidic environment. If we maintain an alkaline environment in our body, it tends to oxygenate the cells that reduce the cancer cell count. Some studies have found that an alkaline environment may make certain chemotherapy drugs more effective or less toxic.

An acidic environment in the body leads to slower metabolism and lesser oxygen in the body. Since oxygen breeds in an alkaline body pH, it creates an atmosphere conducive to losing fat. The higher the oxygen, the better the fat combustion and absorption of nutrients. One of the best things we can do to correct an acidic body is to clean up our diet and lifestyle. Our diet should consist of 60 per cent alkaline-forming foods and 40 per cent acid-forming foods in order to maintain optimal health. To restore one's health and reverse the damage caused by an acidic body, the diet should consist of 80 per cent alkaline-forming foods and 20 per cent acid-forming foods. Incorporating alkaline foods such as lemon water, cucumber, apple cider vinegar, wheatgrass, aloe vera, pumpkin seeds, sunflower seeds, green vegetables like bottle gourd and broccoli, etc. at regular intervals during the day is important to maintain an alkaline body.

We believe in starting the day with a glass of lemon water and cinnamon powder to get rid of morning acidity. Lemon water an hour after every meal will bring the body pH back to alkaline after a typically acidic meal. Lemon water immediately after a meal is not recommended as we need digestive acids to be released in the stomach to enable digestion.

Hacks to keep the body alkaline:

1. Cucumbers and celery are extremely alkaline because of their high water content.

2. Leafy greens (kale, collards, spinach, chard), wheatgrass, sprouts and micro-greens are also quite good because they help increase the amount of oxygen that blood can absorb.

3. Cruciferous vegetables such as broccoli, cauliflower, cabbage and Brussels sprouts provide sulphur to the body.

4. Packed with antioxidants, flavour makers like turmeric, black pepper, ginger, star anise, cinnamon, etc. also help keep your pH in check and strengthen your immune system.

5. The point of alkalizing is to introduce more oxygen into the body, and breathing deeply and consciously will do just that, while making any other steps you try more effective.

Look Beyond Cravings

'I am craving chocolate!' 'I want to eat fries!' 'I feel like having an ice cream!'

While hunger is governed by the stomach, cravings arise in the brain. On some level, hunger is a survival mechanism, but cravings imply your body's communication with you. Haven't we all craved for chocolates or sweets or pasta at some point?

So, What Does It Mean When You are Craving a Particular Food?

It depends on what you are craving for. If you crave chocolate, this means your body needs magnesium and chromium, and not something sweet. Ideally, when we are stressed or fatigued, we have a craving for chocolate, but it's the magnesium that helps our body reduce stress levels and release the 'happiness hormone'. That's why chocolate is known as comfort food.

However, we can always pick a 70 per cent dark chocolate. Sometimes cravings can be more than just a nutrient deficiency. I'd like to share with you a small dialogue:

Tamannaah: Luke, I was shooting in Jaipur and suddenly I had a craving to eat something spicy. I wanted to have green chillies! Long, dark green chillies! However, this was surprising not only to me but the entire crew as this unusual craving popped up on a summer afternoon in Jaipur where the temperature was around 45°C.

Luke: It is completely normal! Like you said, the temperature was extreme, so this is your body's way of signalling that it needs to cool off. Strange, right? Have you noticed that spicy food makes you sweat? Capsaicin, the active chemical in chilli peppers, can induce thermogenesis, the process by which cells convert energy into heat. So, eating chilli increases your metabolism making you sweat more, thereby helping you cool down. Also, eating something with spice helps release endorphins, the good hormone. Maybe your body wanted that high and hence the craving.

Tamannaah: Now I can say, chilli chills you! The body has a beautiful way of sending signals if something is not right, you just need to listen to it.

Like we mentioned earlier, sometimes, cravings indicate that your body needs a particular nutrient. We don't need to consume the food we are craving for, but try instead to figure out what is missing, the cause of the craving. Knowing this will help you replenish the nutrients. You will find additional information about other types of cravings in the food craving chart below, giving you a hint about your cravings. Replenish your nutrients!

If you crave	You need	Foods that satisfy your craving
Chocolate	Magnesium	Raw nuts and seeds, legumes, fruits
Sweets	Chromium	Broccoli, grapes, cheese, dried beans
	Carbon	Fresh fruits
	Phosphorus	Fish, eggs, dairy, nuts, legumes
	Sulphur	Cranberries, horseradish, cruciferous vegetables, kale, cabbage
	Tryptophan	Cheese, lamb, raisins, sweet potato, spinach
Bread/Toast	Nitrogen	High protein foods
Oily Snacks, Fatty Foods	Calcium	Mustard and turnip greens, broccoli, kale, legumes, cheese, sesame
Coffee/Tea	Phosphorus	Beef, liver, poultry, fish, eggs, dairy, nuts, legumes
	Sulphur	Egg yolks, red peppers, muscle protein, garlic, onion, cruciferous vegetables
	Salt	Sea salt, apple cider vinegar
	Iron	Meat, fish and poultry, seaweed, greens, black cherries

Alcohol, Recreational Drugs	Protein	Meat, poultry, seafood, nuts
	Avenin	Steel cut oats
	Calcium	Mustard and turnip greens, broccoli, kale, legumes, cheese, sesame
	Glutamine	Supplements glutamine powder, raw cabbage juice
	Potassium	Sun-dried black olives, potato peel broth, seaweed, bitter greens
Chewing Ice	Iron	Meat, fish and poultry, seaweed, greens, black cherries
Burnt Food	Carbon	Fresh fruits
Soda and Carbonation	Calcium	Mustard and turnip greens, broccoli, kale, legumes, cheese, sesame
Salty Foods	Chloride	Raw goat milk, fish, unrefined sea salt
Acid Foods	Magnesium	Raw nuts and seeds, legumes, fruits
Preference for Liquids rather than Solids	Water	Flavour water with lemon or limes
Cool Drinks	Manganese	Walnuts, almonds, pecans, pineapple, blueberries
Menstrual Cravings	Zinc	Seafood, leafy veggies, root veggies

Overeating	Silicon	Nuts, seeds, avoid refined starches
	Tryptophan	Cheese, lamb, raisins, sweet potato, spinach
	Tyrosine	Vitamin C supplements, or orange, green, red fruits and veggies

Hacks to Combat Constipation

Constipation may be due to the slow movement of food through the digestive system. This may be caused by poor diet, dehydration, medications, chronic illness and diseases affecting the nervous system or some mental disorders. Constipation is not a disease. Constipation may be characterized as passing stools less than three times a week. For some people, constipation may occur rarely while for others it may be a chronic condition. It may refer to lumpy or hard stools, difficulty or unable to pass stools and a sensation of incomplete evacuation. Being constipated can be frustrating and uncomfortable at the same time. Some dietary changes and lifestyle modifications can regularize your bowel movements. If these do not help you should consult a doctor.

1. Add roughage to meals. Both soluble and insoluble fibre are necessary for the smooth functioning of the intestinal system. Most plant foods contain a type of fibre. You should include foods containing a high amount of soluble fibre in your diet like oatmeal, potatoes, dried beans, rice bran, barley, citrus fruits and peas. Avoid junk, processed foods, cheese, meat and ice creams as much as possible.

2. Break free from a sedentary lifestyle and move more.

3. Handle emotions in a better way since the gut and brain are closely connected.

4. Clear your bowels around the same time every day.

5. Keep your body well hydrated.

Lastly, some natural remedies that address constipation:

- Psyllium husk or isabgul is a natural laxative, much better than a synthetic one. It works well for those who are chronically constipated or travel a lot. 2–3 tsp of this mixed with water can lead to a smoother motion the next morning.

- 1 tbsp of triphala powder mixed with water before bed helps clean the colon the next day.

- Eat 4–5 soaked prunes/2 tbsp black raisins/dried apricots with warm water, 2 hours before bed.

- Soak ½ tsp of ajwain in hot water and drink to stimulate the motions.

- 1 tbsp of castor oil/extra virgin coconut oil before bed helps lubricate the passage.

The takeaway message: When it comes to immunity, detoxification and overall good health, there is no place for constipation at all. It is a serious issue because everything depends on the way you expel toxic waste from the colon. Not only do you prevent a disease, but also manage and heal in a better way.

Hacks to Combat Acidity

There are so many people today who suffer from acid reflux, acidity, burping, bloating and flatulence. These are all forms of acidity, which if not handled properly and at the right time, can cause innumerable ailments like cancer, diabetes, poor skin quality, inability to lose weight, poor hair quality and other ailments.

Every cell in your body requires oxygen to remain healthy. In an acidic body, these cells become anaerobic which means they don't allow oxygen to reach the cells completely. So when your cells are deprived of oxygen, the body starts facing problems and diseases. These are simple lifestyle changes that can help you get rid of even the most serious cases of acidity.

Let's get rid of certain factors that may cause acid reflux. These include:

- Excessive consumption of alcohol
- Smoking
- Prolonged fasting
- Chronic stress
- Extremely spicy food
- Frequent intake of non-vegetarian food
- Medicines, e.g. Non-Steroidal Anti-Inflammatory Drugs (NSAIDs)
- H. Pylori infection R

Remedies to combat acidity:

1. Maintain a gap of 3.5–4 hours (max) between each meal. Consuming meals too frequently is not a good idea as well (as frequently as 2–2.5 hours). It compels the body to produce acid frequently to break down the food coming infrequently.

2. Minimize the intake of pickles, spicy chutneys and other preserved and processed foods.

3. It is important to remain upright for at least 2 hours after eating every meal.

4. Make sure you don't overeat.

5. Avoid lying down after a large meal as this may lead to acid reflux.

6. While sleeping, raise the pillow to a 40 degree angle or by 6 to 8 inches, to avoid flux.

7. Wear loose clothing, especially at night.

8. Ensure adequate hydration throughout the day. Keep the water intake at 2.5 to 3 litres a day. Sip on it at frequent intervals, space it out well. Avoid drinking too much at a time and avoid drinking water during meals.

9. Sucking on a piece of clove is another effective remedy.

10. Eat cucumber in salads or by itself.

11. Have 1 banana every day (have two if there is excess discomfort).

12. Add basil leaves to salad or soup or simply chew them.

13. When you eat in stress, you are bound to invite acidity. Make sure you take 6–10 long deep breaths right before a meal; this will ensure the shift in the system from sympathetic to parasympathetic (rest and digest). Also eat the food absolutely slowly, take about 20 minutes to eat the food without gadgets or any diversions.

14. Make a drink of ajwain, saunf and jeera with some warm water/lemon water. Both ajwain and saunf have been popular because they aid digestion. Consume this 30–45 minutes after your meals.

Hacks to Combat Diarrhoea

Diarrhoea is the condition of having three or more loose or liquid bowel movements in a day. The loss of fluids during loose motions can cause dehydration and electrolyte disturbances. Signs of dehydration often begin with loss of the normal stretchiness of the skin and changes in personality. This can progress to decreased urination, loss of skin colour, quicker heart rate, and a decrease in responsiveness as it becomes more severe.

Sometimes stress or anxiety can also cause diarrhoea. The reason that you can experience diarrhoea when you are stressed is directly related to your body's programmed stress response, what is commonly referred to as our fight-or-flight reaction. When your body is in overdrive, it causes a surge of adrenaline to redistribute your blood flow to safeguard your key organs. This means that blood flows more to your brain, heart, lungs and muscles. During this time, your gut does not receive as much blood flow as it normally would, leading to poor stool health and intestines that are processing food improperly. Address the root cause and let's work on it. Deep breathing, meditation, yoga can help.

Remedies:

1. Soluble fibre helps when there's a diarrhoeal attack. This fibre soaks up liquid in the intestine and forms a gel. This gel reduces the peristaltic movement of the intestine which in turn reduces the gastric emptying time that helps to stop or slow down diarrhoea. Good sources of soluble fibre include beans, oats and some fruits such as apples, bananas, oranges, sweet limes, strawberries and grapefruit.

2. 1 tbsp arrowroot powder in a glass of water.

3. Black tea/Black coffee with lemon.

4. Stay hydrated. Oral rehydration solutions, lemon water with salt, buttermilk with salt, coconut water are some good options to replenish loss of electrolytes.

5. Diarrhoea drains away good bacteria that helps prevent harmful bacteria from growing out of control. Natural probiotics like yoghurt and buttermilk can help alleviate diarrhoea. However, it is essential for the person to take a probiotic supplement.

Hacks to Combat Bloating

Are you one who wakes up to a huge round belly and a puffy face in the morning that soon settles down towards midday, and come evening you regain the puffiness once again? And just because of how you felt in the morning, you have cursed yourself all day long, and even punished your body by going on a starvation diet?

Well, what if you are not fat, but just bloated?

Most of us tend to confuse the two. There is a huge difference between being fat and being bloated. Fat is the accumulation of fat cells in the body due to improper diet, lack of activity, inadequate sleep and stress. Bloating on the other hand is experienced due to the accumulation of either a lot of fluids or gases within the body.

Why does the body retain water in the first place? The main factor that triggers water retention is a wrong lifestyle.

1. If you find yourself sitting in one place for prolonged periods of time, you are inviting water retention because of poor circulation and pooling of blood in a specific area.

2. Chemotherapy drugs, beta blockers, antidepressants and NSAIDS cause water retention as a side effect.

3. Lack of sleep leading to hormonal imbalance.

4. Chronic stress, emotional imbalance, emotional internalization.

5. Exceeding the daily limit of salt intake by eating processed foods.

6. High intake of sugar and other junk food.

7. Medical conditions like a sluggish liver, poor kidney health and weak heart health are all linked to water retention.

Ways to beat bloating? Popping diuretics like lasix is not the solution. It can compromise the health of our kidneys in the long run and create an imbalance in normal levels of electrolytes that are vital to heart, kidney and liver functions. If the root cause is lifestyle, then the solution should revolve around lifestyle, too.

Quick Remedies:

1. Natural foods like parsley and coriander work as fantastic natural diuretics. Take about 250 gm of each and keep boiling them in water till it loses its colour. Strain the yellowish liquid and keep sipping on it all day.

2. Boil 1 tbsp of fennel seeds and 1 tsp of bishops weed in 4 cups of water, reduce to half, strain and sip.

3. Boil 3 tbsp of pearl barley in 3 cups of water, reduce to half, and add some lemon juice.

4. Soak 1 tbsp of coriander seeds overnight in 1 glass of water. In the morning, strain and sip the water.

5. Magnesium is responsible for carrying out more than 300 enzymatic functions including balancing the right amount of sodium. Almonds, bananas, whole grains and cacao nibs are some of the best sources.

6. A combination of black sesame seeds and jaggery is known to reduce menstruation-related bloating.

7. Just like magnesium, potassium balances excess sodium. Bananas, tomatoes, avocadoes, nuts, and seeds are potassium-rich sources.

Hacks to Combat Anaemia

Anaemia is a medical condition in which the red blood cell (RBC) count or haemoglobin is less than normal. For men, anaemia is typically defined as a haemoglobin level of less than 13.5 gm/100 ml and in women as haemoglobin of less than 12.0 gm/100 ml. There are more than 400 types of anaemia.

Anaemia is caused by either a decrease in production of RBCs or haemoglobin or an increase in loss (usually due to bleeding) or increased destruction of RBCs.

The line of treatment:

1. Consider a diet that includes good sources of iron, vitamin B12, and folate. Ensure you combine iron-rich sources with a vitamin C-rich source for better iron absorption.

2. A glass of wheatgrass juice with lemon/amla.

3. 1 tsp of moringa powder in a glass of lemon water. If you find fresh moringa leaves, you can juice them, too.

4. Include these sources in your diet: broccoli, spinach, dill, drumstick, eggs and chicken liver.

5. Examples of folic acid-rich food sources: Beans and lentils, dark green leafy vegetables like spinach, collard or turnip greens, cruciferous vegetables (cauliflower, broccoli, cabbage), okra, Brussels sprouts and asparagus. Cooking the vegetables helps get rid of phytates.

6. Avoid having calcium and iron sources together as they compete for the same carrier for absorption.

7. Have 2–3 dates daily.

8. A simple glass of lemon water with 1 tbsp of jaggery will also help combat anaemia.

9. A juice of kulekhara leaves with a few drops of lemon is also very effective.

10. A glass of beetroot juice with ginger and lemon.

11. Ensure you mix an iron-rich source with vitamin C-rich food for better absorption. Sources of vitamin C: Amla, lemon, orange, kiwi, sweet lime, etc.

Hacks to Prevent the Greying of Hair

Hair primarily turns grey when melanocytes around the hair follicles decrease or stop production of melanin. Grey strands of hair are a person's most devastating nightmare. Keratin is the main protein that builds hair. The absence or deficiency of melanin in keratin causes hair greying. Deficiency of melanin can be caused by genetics, age and hormonal changes in the body. Chemical dyes to blacken hair and redeem hair's lustre and shine may have harmful effects in the long run. So here, we talk about some natural remedies which can help turn grey hair to black.

1. Applying black tea to your grey hair can gradually make your hair black. It also helps increase the volume of hair and makes hair shinier. Use the black tea mask twice a week and avoid using a shampoo after this treatment for effective results.

2. Both coconut oil and lemon are great ingredients for your hair. They help in preserving pigment cells in hair follicles and make hair blacker, day by day.

3. Amla is great for the hair and has proven to be even more beneficial when you use it as dye paste. You can mix amla juice with henna and apply it to your hair. A combination of amla and henna is probably the best home remedy to cure greyness. Apply the pack once a month for effective results.

4. You can make a really easy potato mask at home which will blacken your hair gradually, but effectively. All you have to do is boil a potato until the starch solution begins to form. Use the strained liquid from the potato peels and apply it to your hair. Rinse it off with water. The starch solution from potatoes helps restore hair pigment and prevents greying.

5. You just have to boil a ribbed gourd, add coconut oil and apply when the solution has cooled down. This pack helps strengthen hair roots. Apply this mask two or three times a week for effective results.

6. Oats are popular for their numerous health benefits, but did you know that they can also turn grey hair black?

Prepare a paste of oats by adding almond oil. The rich presence of biotin in oats proves to be a great healer of grey hair.

7. Onion juice has been found to be rich in catalase, an enzyme responsible for darkening hair from the roots. Onion juice is a good source of biotin, magnesium, copper, vitamin C, phosphorus, sulphur, vitamins B1 and B6, and folate. These help blacken your hair and also help prevent hair fall. To make an onion pack, all you have to do is extract juice from an onion and apply it on your hair, particularly on the roots. Leave the pack for 40 minutes and rinse off. This pack can be applied twice a week for effective results.

Hacks to Reduce Mucositis (Mouth Sores)

1. Do oil pulling or chew a piece of dried coconut (one inch).

2. Gargle with warm water containing salt and turmeric.

3. Apply a paste made of pure turmeric powder and organic raw honey over the sores. Leave it for 20–30 minutes. Then, wash it off.

4. Apply a paste of baking soda and water over the sores. Leave it for 20–30 minutes. Then, wash it off.

5. Make sure you consume easy-to-swallow and soft food items.

6. Avoid too hot, too cold, or very spicy and acidic food items.

Hacks for Nausea and Vomiting

1. Take slow sips from a glass of lemon water (about ½ lemon squeezed in 200–250 ml of water); or lick a lemon wedge.

2. Chew 4–5 fresh clean mint leaves.

3. Suck 1–2 holy basil leaves.

4. Chew 1–2 pods of cardamom.

5. Consume a mixture containing 1 tsp of fresh ginger juice with 1 tsp of fresh lemon juice in 1 cup of water.

6. Take 2 drops of peppermint oil or lavender oil and apply it gently over the temples and nostrils, and breathe in the aroma.

7. Chew ½ tsp cumin seeds.

Hacks for Loss of Appetite

1. Consume a mixture containing 1 tsp of fresh ginger juice with 1 tsp of fresh lemon juice in 1 cup of water, 30 minutes before meals.

2. Chew on a gooseberry, or drink fresh gooseberry juice (made using 2–3 amlas).

3. Drink 1 cup of fresh coriander juice (take a handful of clean and organic coriander leaves and blend them with water).

4. Chew ½ tsp of roasted cumin seeds.

Hacks for Body Aches and Pains

1. Epsom salt (magnesium sulphate) soak:

    Add 50–100 g of Epsom salt in a bucket of warm water and soak your legs up to the knees for 10–15 minutes.

    Hydrate yourself after the soak with 1–2 glasses of water as this soak tends to dehydrate you a little.

    Note: People with low blood pressure may need to avoid this soak.

2. Nutmeg-sesame oil application:

   Take 4–5 drops of pure nutmeg essential oil and mix it with ¼ cup of pure sesame oil.

   Gently apply and massage this oil on the aching area.

   Keep it overnight for a better effect.

3. Sesame oil or coconut oil and camphor mix:

   Warm up about ¼ cup of coconut or sesame oil and combine it with a few pieces of camphor. Massage this mixture around the aching area.

   Keep it overnight for a better effect.

4. Hot compress or hot and cold compress alternately can also help.

5. Keep a check on your serum vitamins D3, B12 and magnesium levels.

Hacks to Reduce Pigmentation

1. Raw potato juice application:

   Take a raw potato and wash it thoroughly. Remove the green offshoots, if any.

   Chop it into pieces and blend in a mixer with a little water to form a paste. Apply it on the affected area and leave it for 30 minutes.

   Then, wash it off with plain water. Pat the area dry.

   Now, apply cold-pressed virgin coconut oil over the area.

2. Aloe vera gel application:

   Apply fresh aloe vera gel over the affected area.

   It helps reduce pigmentation and also soothes the skin.

3. Cold-pressed virgin coconut oil application:

Apply cold-pressed virgin coconut oil over the affected area regularly. This will help reduce pigmentation.

4. Consume liquorice tea.

5. Scrub your face with this DIY scrub: Mix 1 tsp turmeric, 1 cup gram flour, milk or water to smoothen the mixture.

6. Apply tomato juice on your face for 30 minutes and wash it off.

7. Mix amla powder in almond milk and apply on your face for 30 minutes and wash it off.

8. Mix 1 tbsp apple cider vinegar with mother culture in 4 tbsp water and use this mixture to cleanse your face regularly.

9. Take 1 tbsp of orange peel powder, 1 tbsp of multani mitti and make a smooth paste by adding rose water. Apply on face and rinse off only when it's semi-dry.

10. Mix 1 tbsp pomegranate peel powder with 1 tbsp milk and apply on your face like a face pack.

11. Apply mashed papaya mixed with fresh cream on your face for 1 hour and wash off.

12. Apply apple juice mixed with curd on your face for 45 minutes and wash it off.

Hacks to Reduce Fever/Body Temperature

1. Fenugreek seeds water: Take 1 tbsp of fenugreek seeds; boil it in 300 ml of water. Reduce it to 150–200 ml and sip it warm twice daily.

2. Keep a cold compress over the forehead.

3. Cover the feet by wearing cotton socks.

Hacks for Common Cold

Most of us have suffered from common cold but the real question here is, how fast did you recover? Did you take any medicine to recover?

More often than not, we turn to medical advice that provides short-term relief. Unfortunately, most cough syrups and cough drops on the market provide little relief and don't treat the cause of the problem. Using home remedies for cough that actually deal with the cause of the symptom is crucial while fighting infections, to thin mucus and boost your immune system.

When you can't seem to get rid of a cough, there are a few food items that can help thin mucus, soothe your muscles, reduce inflammation and boost your immune system. The natural home remedies for cough are as follows:

1. Luke's Magic Potion: 1 inch ginger (mashed), 1 clove garlic, 3 peppercorns, 2 cloves, 2 cardamoms, 1 cinnamon stick; boil and reduce to half, strain, add organic honey (1 tbsp), sip it hot.

2. Luke's Magic Lung Tea: 1 inch ginger or ½ tsp dried ginger powder, 1 small Sri Lankan rolled cinnamon stick, ½ tsp basil leaves (fresh/dry), ½ tsp oregano (fresh/dry), 1 peppercorn, 2 crushed elaichis (optional: 1 or 2 crushed garlic cloves), 1 tbsp fennel seeds, a pinch of ajwain, ¼ tsp cumin seeds). Boil for 10 minutes, let it simmer.

3. Water: Start by drinking plenty of water throughout the day, 3 litres per day. This will help thin the mucus that's building up in your airways and causing a cough.

4. Bone broth: Sipping on real bone broth can support your immunity, thin mucus in your airways, soothe your muscles, and promote detoxification. When your cough is caused by exposure to toxins, chemicals, pesticides or

artificial ingredients that are causing an inflammatory reaction, consuming bone broth can be helpful in removing those substances from your body.

5. Raw garlic: Allicin, a compound found in garlic, is known for its ability to kill microorganisms that are responsible for respiratory infections that can lead to coughing. Raw garlic has antimicrobial, antiviral and antifungal properties, so adding it to your diet as a natural cough remedy can be beneficial in helping you get rid of infection.

6. Ginger tea: Drinking ginger tea when you have a cough can help boost your immune system and fight the infection that's causing the symptom. Ginger root benefits come from its powerful antibacterial, antiviral and antifungal properties, which makes it perfect when dealing with respiratory tract infections.

7. Probiotic foods: One possible side effect of not having enough probiotics is frequent colds and coughs, because probiotics are responsible for supporting your immune system. To fight your cough, try eating probiotic foods like cultured vegetables, rice kanji, beetroot kanji, sauerkraut and kimchi, coconut kefir, apple cider vinegar, miso and kombucha.

8. In an effort to reduce inflammation and mucus production, avoid consuming sweetened beverages, fruit juices, sugary foods, chocolate, processed foods and conventional dairy products when you have a cough. Instead of drinking juice or sweetened drinks, choose whole fruits and vegetables instead, that are much higher in vitamin C and will help boost your immune function.

9. Vitamin C can be used as a home remedy for cough because it supports your immune system and boosts your white blood cells. Vitamin C also serves as an

important antioxidant that may help reduce cough and wheezing in smokers who have high levels of oxidative stress.

10. Essential oils can help loosen your mucus, relax the muscles of your respiratory system and allow more oxygen to reach your lungs. Some of the best essential oils for cough are eucalyptus, peppermint and lemon.

Hacks for Sinusitis

1. Application of eucalyptus oil on the bridge of nostril.

2. Warm compression using towel over the sinus area.

3. Apply dry ginger paste around the bridge of your nose.

4. Steam inhalation using 3–4 drops of peppermint oil/ eucalyptus oil and 1 tsp turmeric powder.

5. Use a castor oil pack on the chest: Warm a cup of cold pressed castor oil, dip a cotton cloth into and wring out the oil. Place the cloth on the pain area and put a hot water bag or heating pad on top for around 10 minutes.

6. Consume 1 tbsp horseradish with lemon.

7. Adequate hydration is the key to flushing out the virus and hence sinusitis.

8. Consume ginger, garlic, lemon.

Hacks to Combat Seasonal Allergies

1. Anti-allergy drink: Blend ½ tsp amla, 1 tsp aloe vera, ½ tsp turmeric, a pinch of black pepper, 1 inch ginger, 1 tsp tulsi, ¼ tsp neem powder, 1 tsp jaggery in 100 ml water and consume.

2. Consume 1 clove of honey soaked garlic daily.

3. Drink 2–3 glasses of lemon water to help detoxify the body.

4. Add a probiotic like rice kanji, kombucha, beetroot kanji, yoghurt, etc. to your diet.

5. Drink a glass of water with a teaspoon of apple cider vinegar with mother culture.

6. Add quercetin-rich foods that fight against allergies; cabbage, cauliflower, broccoli, onions/shallots, green tea, citrus fruits, etc.

7. Try practicing a yogic cleansing technique called *jalneti*.

8. Have 1 cup nettle leaf tea.

Hacks to Reduce Ear Pain

Home-Made Ear Drops and Remedies that Work Wonders:

The recipes mentioned below are for applying drops in the affected ear using a clean dropper bottle or baby syringe. Cover your ear with a cotton ball or clean cloth, and lean on the opposite side to allow the drops to enter and sit in the ear. Do this for about 5 minutes. In case you feel any uneasiness, flip over to the other side, and let the mixture drain out.

1. Holy basil ear drops: Blend a handful of tulsi leaves, and boil it for 5 minutes in 2 cups water. Reduce it to half, then strain by pressing the extract, and allow it to cool. Using a dropper, you can put 2–3 drops of this in the affected ear.

2. Onion juice ear drops: Chop one onion, and boil in 100 ml water. Reduce it to half, cool, strain, and put 2–3 drops of this extracted juice in the affected ear for 5 minutes.

3. Garlic–sesame oil ear drops: Sauté garlic in 1 tbsp of cold-pressed sesame oil. Let it cool. Carefully take only the oil and add 2–3 drops to the affected ear (garlic–mustard oil combination also works, but first, try a tiny drop, and observe your tolerance).

4. Mustard ear drops: Heat cold-pressed mustard oil, and let it cool. Put 1–2 drops of this oil into the ear.

5. Ginger ear drops: Apply warm ginger juice around the outer ear canal (outer application only).

6. Olive oil ear drops: Putting a few drops of warm olive oil in the ear helps, too.

7. Oregano ear drops: Heat 1 tsp of oregano with 2 tbsp of cold-pressed coconut oil, and leave it overnight. Strain and apply 2–3 drops of this oil in the ear.

8. Tea tree oil ear drops: Mix 2–3 drops of tea tree oil with 1 tsp of olive oil, and place 2–3 drops inside the ear.

9. Clove–sesame oil ear drops: Sauté 2 cloves in 1 tbsp of cold-pressed sesame oil. Apply 2–3 drops of this inside the ear.

10. Ajwain ear drops: Heat 1 tsp of ajwain with cold-pressed coconut or sesame oil, and leave it overnight. Strain and apply 2–3 drops of this oil in the ear

11. Apple cider vinegar ear drops: Mix apple cider vinegar with mother and water in a 1:3 ratio. Apply 3–4 drops in each affected ear.

12. For babies: A drop of breast milk in each ear helps.

13. Neem juice: 2–3 drops of strained neem juice extracted by crushing the leaves, or dip a cotton swab in neem oil, squeeze out the excess, and then place it in your ear for a few minutes before removing it.

14. Peeled garlic: Place peeled garlic (big) near the affected ear for 15–20 minutes. Ensure the garlic does not slip into the ear.

15. Sleep posture: Sleep with the affected ear raised, instead of having it face down on the pillow. This can help the ear drain better if necessary.

16. Music therapy: Music and sound therapy also work well.

17. Ice or warm compress: Place an ice pack or a warm compress over the ear, and alternate between warm and cold for 10 minutes.

18. Sweet almond oil: Take warm sweet almond oil, and massage it in at the point where your ear joins your cheek. You could also use olive oil or mustard oil instead of almond oil.

19. Garlic and ajwain mix: Heat some garlic and ajwain on a pan. Place it in a cloth, and make a warm compress for the ear; this can be done for kids; too.

20. Hair dry: Use a hairdryer on low to dry the water from the ears after washing your hair.

Hacks to Handle Vertigo

While medicines to cure vertigo do exist, one must also invest time and effort to find out what has caused this ailment. Parallel lifestyle changes to reduce dependency on medications is a good way to go. Lifestyle change can also help lessen the severity of vertigo and also help regain balance.

Some lifestyle measures that should be followed include:

1. Ginger juice: This has long been one of the most effective home remedies for vertigo. It helps immensely in reducing inflammation. One can add a tsp of fresh ginger juice in water or vegetable juice before consuming.

2. Anti-inflammatory foods: Anti-inflammatory foods such as turmeric, pepper, cayenne pepper, garlic and cumin seeds should be included as part of the diet.

3. Jerky movements: Avoiding jerky movements and immediately getting up from a sleeping position. Turn on one side and get up slowly. Avoid bending forward.

4. Hydration and electrolyte balance: Improve water intake and electrolyte balance. Coconut water and lemon water

with a pinch of pink salt helps to a great extent. Lemon water also helps in keeping the body alkaline.

5. Fresh mint or basil leaves: Chewing fresh mint or basil leaves helps combat associated nausea, vomiting and even headaches. One can even explore ginger and peppermint essential oils.

6. Stress: Manage stress effectively; increased stress leads to an increase in inflammation and affects sleep, too. Deep breathing, early dinners, journaling, herbal teas like chamomile, lemongrass and lavender help promote sleep.

7. Gut health: Improve your gut health by cutting down potent irritants like sugar, caffeine, milk and wheat. Instead, include foods like papaya and pineapple that are rich in digestive enzymes.

8. Proper posture: Maintain an upright posture. Cut down time spent on gadgets and electronic devices. Hold the phone parallel to your eye line to avoid bending your neck.

9. Vitamin B12: Boost vitamin B12 levels, if they are low. B12 is associated with neurological health as well as feeling off-balance.

10. Get fresh air if you can, or open a window.

11. Conscious and controlled breathing has immense positive effects on vertigo. Pranayama helps infuse every cell with oxygen, including the brain, and also calms the nervous system. Anulom vilom, left nostril breathing, and bhramari breathing are highly recommended. *Balasana*, *shavasana*, *viparita karani* and *supta baddha konasana* (preferably under expert guidance) are a few recommended asanas.

12. Practicing *shanmukhi mudra* also helps a lot.

13. Sound-producing breaths like bhramari and omkar chanting helps calm the nervous system and produces

vibrations in the body that are extremely relaxing and positive.

Hacks to Stay Warm in Winter

Add the following foods to warm up your winter:

1. Ghee: Pure and ethically sourced A2 ghee is one of the most easily digestible immunity-boosting fats that generates instant heat and energy to keep your body warm. We can change our cooking medium to ghee or add it to your roti, rice, or khichdi during the winter season. It also keeps the skin moist and prevents dryness associated with winters.

2. Amla: The Indian gooseberry comes packed with immunity-boosting vitamin C that helps keep infections at bay. You can have amla in the form of murabba, pickles, candies, chutneys, juice, or eat the fruit with a sprinkle of black pepper powder.

3. Chikki (peanut brittle): Winter is the season to eat chikki or traditional energy bars. A lot of commercially bought chikki is loaded with liquid glucose, white sugar and maltodextrin. You can make chikki at home with sesame seeds or peanuts and jaggery. Chikki generates good heat in the body. Sesame seeds are a rich source of calcium, zinc, manganese, and even iron to keep the bones strong and ensure healthy blood circulation. During winters, it is vital to maintain adequate iron levels, as iron aids in binding oxygen to RBCs. Lower the amount of iron, lesser the availability of oxygen in the body, and the colder you feel. The beauty of Indian culture is that chikki is also served as a traditional food during festivals like Lohri and Makar Sankranti.

4. Bajra (pearl millet) and maize flour: Maize flour and bajra tops the charts when it comes to warming foods. These foods are fibre-rich starches that provide energy, increase blood circulation, and hence raise the body temperature. One can make rotis, laddoos, crackers, or millet khichdi with ghee.

5. Panjiri: This dry and sweet snack prepared during winters in the northern parts of our country is very warming and believed to help relieve body pains and open up muscles and joints. One can make different versions of this using whole wheat, millets, sattu, or moong dal flour; to this, add ghee, nuts, dry fruits, and spices like cardamom, fennel seeds, saffron and nutmeg.

6. Fresh turmeric root: It is an anti-bacterial, anti-inflammatory, anti-viral, anti-fungal, and a significant warming food that helps stimulate your immune system. Have 1 tsp of this with salt and lemon, or add it to pickles or turmeric milk.

7. Fresh green garlic: We call it a natural antibiotic because of its allicin content which is a potent disease-fighting food. We know it is anti-inflammatory and of high medicinal value, and hence it is imperative to add it to your diet. One can prepare chutney of green garlic with coriander leaves and consume with meals or have it steamed.

8. Ginger–Honey: The mixture of good quality ginger juice and raw unpasteurized honey will keep your body warm and prevent mucus formation. 1 tbsp of this mixture on an empty stomach is a good idea.

9. Leafy greens: They are a potent nutritional powerhouse, abundant in phytochemicals, vitamins and minerals. The Indian dishes sarson ka saag and undhiyu are a great blend of traditional wisdom meant to be relished during winter months.

10. Laddoo: Winter is the time to consume all sorts of laddoos like methi/guar gum/urad dal/dry fruits/dates. All these are winter superfoods—warming and energizing! You can increase the protein content by adding sattu, and as long as we add jaggery to it, it is good to go, as jaggery is a warming food and perfect for winters.

11. Guar gum: This looks like a hard raisin and is great winter food. It is fluffed in ghee and then consumed by adding it in laddoos, panjiri or by itself. It is excellent for improving strength and lubrication in bones.

12. Raab/Porridge: This can be prepared with ragi or bajra. Having a warm bowl of raab is hugely beneficial, as it keeps the body warm and prevents mucous formation.

13. Root vegetables: Sweet potatoes, yam, turnips and carrots are loaded with beta-carotene which is a source of vitamin A, good fibre, potassium and manganese, most of the B vitamins and many more nutrients.

14. Kadha: Kadha or herbal concoction is the way to go in winters. Take some carom seeds, cumin seeds, fennel, Ceylon cinnamon, black pepper, tulsi, and prepare a magical concoction! You can add some ginger for its throat-relieving properties and raw honey for sweetness.

15. Green peas: Our much loved tender green peas flood the markets in winters. They are rich in folate and protein and make a perfect winter food.

16. Tulsi: This inexpensive, easy-to-grow and a widely found herb/adaptogen has multiple health benefits, from fighting bacterial and viral infections to strengthening your immune system, especially in winters.

17. Fresh seasonal berries: Ensure you consume the seasonal produce and berries like strawberries and litchis. They are abundant in the winter season and are perfect for immunity.

18. Jaggery: Good quality, ethically sourced jaggery is an iron-rich sweetener. It soothes throat irritation by creating a layer on the inner lining of our throat, provides a soothing sensation and reduces dryness. It also dilates the blood vessels, improves blood flow, and produces warmth in the body.

19. Garden cress seeds: Garden cress seeds contain a host of nutrients. They are loaded with iron and are also an excellent source of folic acid, vitamins C, A and E, dietary fibre, calcium, protein, and most importantly, help increase body heat. Soak 1 tsp of these seeds and add it to your smoothies or laddoos, or have it with lemon water.

20. Saffron: Add this underutilized yet effective spice to warm up your winter. You can have it with milk or porridge or rice or laddoos or any sweet.

Hacks to Combat Summer Heat

Add the following foods to cool the system:

1. Fennel seeds can be chewed or had as a juice.

2. Bael can be eaten or turned into a drink.

3. Kokum can be added to curries or consumed as a juice or consider having sol kadhi.

4. Sabja can be soaked for 4–5 hours and then had by adding it to water or juice.

5. Cumin seeds can be chewed or sprinkled over salad or had in the form of jal jeera.

6. Curd can be consumed as buttermilk or lassi or simply as a snack.

7. Add cucumber to a salad, or make a juice, or have it mid meal.

8. Aam panna.

9. Add mint to salad or water, or have its juice.
10. Green chilli is spicy but it cools the system. You may have 1 small chilli if you are not allergic or have gut issues.
11. Onions.
12. Coconut water.
13. Celery.
14. Prepare a tea made with coriander seeds.
15. Add cilantro to gravies or have it as a juice.
16. Melons.
17. Prepare a syrup of vetiver roots and add 1–2 tbsp in water and enjoy.
18. Suck on a cardamom pod or make some cardamom tea.
19. Have a jowar roti/upma/chilla/dosa/khichdi/porridge
20. Add liquorice to tea or suck a stick.
21. Rosewater can be a midday refresher or you can also make gulkand with dried rose petals.
22. ⅛ tsp of sandalwood can be consumed with milk or water.
23. Amla murabba or juice is a great idea; or chew it or add its powder in water.
24. Lemon water is a refreshing summer drink.

Hacks to Sleep Better

Sleep is one of the most powerful lifestyle drugs that we all need for disease prevention as well as to heal. Some of us are blessed with a good quality of sleep every single day while many of us experience bad quality of sleep. A better way to describe insomnia is when a person faces trouble falling asleep or staying asleep for a longer time despite being tired or sleepy.

Insomnia can trap you in a poor lifestyle circle since all pillars of lifestyle are interlinked. When your sleep is incomplete, you can't function optimally. This affects your quality of work leading to increased stress. You are easily fatigued, workouts are stressful as your body doesn't get enough rest needed for recovery. You feel drowsy, irritated, low, impatient, inactive, unable to concentrate, take time in the simplest of things and it affects your ability to make decisions. Most importantly, when you are sleep-deprived, you crave unhealthy foods that could lead to unnecessary weight gain. Serious sleep disorders could also be linked to hypertension, irregular heartbeat, weak immunity and increase in stress hormone levels. Good sleep helps you to eat better, exercise better and stay healthier.

Good health is all about having equilibrium with all pillars of lifestyle like sleep, stress, food, exercise and water intake. One needs to get to the root cause of not being able to fall asleep which actually is such a natural phenomenon and hence, I would like to discuss the top 15 ways to handle insomnia keeping all those pillars in mind:

1. A heavy meal close to bedtime can make one feel acidic and may cause difficulty falling asleep as metabolism of the body increases when the digestive system is active.

2. Avoid stimulators like caffeine, alcohol, spicy food, tobacco, etc. close to bedtime.

3. Nutmeg is a natural sleep spice being used since ancient times in India. A pinch of nutmeg with water; or a dash of nutmeg, 1 tbsp of fennel, a pinch of cinnamon— boil in water and consume 30 minutes before bedtime. However, too much nutmeg can make you high and acidic.

4. Food rich in amino acid tryptophan will release the sleep hormone melatonin in the body—pumpkin, almonds, organic A2 milk, yoghurt, etc. are good options for bedtime snacking. However, dairy during

bedtime can trouble some people with congestion and hence you can only have it if it suits you.

5. Chlorophyll-rich vegetables like wheatgrass, moringa, barley grass, celery, etc. contain a component called opium that acts as a natural sleeping aid. Consuming them during the daytime is more beneficial than consuming it at bedtime.

6. A warm cup of camomile tea helps calm the body down and aids in better sleep quality.

7. Left nostril breathing will cool the body down internally. Block your right nostril completely along with your mouth, and use your left nostril to inhale and exhale for a couple of rounds. Make sure you're lying down while you're conducting this exercise.

8. 6-6-12 breathing technique helps calm the body instantly. Inhale-Hold-Exhale and repeat for a couple of rounds. You inhale for 6 seconds, hold for 6 seconds and exhale for 12 seconds. Beginners can use the 4-7-8 technique.

9. Aim to meditate, visualize and write affirmations 10–15 minutes before bedtime. This helps reduce the anxiety of not falling asleep on time. For instance, jot down sentences like: I was able to sleep deeply today; I'm embracing the peace and a calm state of mind as I wake up; All my body cells are resting and recovering while I sleep; Sleep is quite natural and I deserve every minute of rest during the night.

10. Irregular or long daytime naps should be avoided as it will make it difficult for your body to fall asleep again at night. However, when you've not had a good night's sleep, taking a nap of 40–60 minutes during the day would be valuable.

11. Ensure a fixed bedtime routine for a sound sleep. It's important to set our biological clock as per the routine.

Changing it occasionally due to social obligations is okay, but making it a lifestyle is something which isn't encouraged.

12. Limit your screen time just before going to bed. Gadgets emit light which blocks melatonin (the sleep hormone). Also, darken the room thirty minutes before bedtime so your brain gets the signal that it's time for you to fall asleep now.

13. Yogasanas like *shirsanana, sarvangasana, uttanasana, viparit karni, paschimotanasana* and *shavala* are helpful for someone dealing with insomnia. *Yoga nidra* and *shawasana* are quite helpful when done during bedtime.

14. A warm shower before bedtime will drop your body temperature a bit that helps you sleep faster. One can also use essential oils or Epsom salt in water which can further relax the nerves and muscles.

15. Go on a holiday once every 6–7 months for a couple of days away from the city's hustle and bustle. Nature is the best healer and it allows the body to heal naturally when exposed to it correctly.

16. Add 1 tbsp poppy seeds to your dinner meal.

17. Sprinkle a few drops of lavender essential oil on the pillow or use a diffuser. All in all, a night of good sleep is a must to heal the mind and body. All the above tips will help you sleep better. However, make sure you're consistent and patient about the changes happening in the body. If you're on any sleep medication, you may want to speak to your doctor before you decide to choose a holistic approach. This way you can avoid any complications that may arise from discontinuing your medication suddenly.

Hacks to Transit into Menopause Smoothly

• Hot flashes and night sweats

This happens due to a hormonal imbalance, and the upper part of a woman's body feels warm and may cause excessive sweating.

Solution:

1. Boil 1 inch ginseng in 2 cups water; steep, strain and drink.
2. Peppermint oil/lavender oil in a diffuser; add 2–3 drops.
3. Niranjan Phal: Soak 2–3 niranjan phal for 30 minutes and consume with skin. If you have a cold or a cough, then peel the skin before consuming.
4. Cotton clothes and cotton undergarments so that air can pass freely and you can feel better.
5. Apply an ice cube on the nape of your neck for instant coolness.
6. 1 tsp sabja in 1 cup water.
7. Fresh rose petals or gulkand (without sweetener), or honey/jaggery; the infused water will cool your body temperature and release heat.
8. Fennel seeds or khus water helps, too.

• Mood swings, irritability, anxiety or depression/sadness/ low self-esteem

Solution:

1. Accept that it will happen.
2. Talk about positive things and you will have positive things in life.
3. Don't fear menopause, as it will be difficult to handle.

4. Manage your stress so that your transition to menopause is smooth. High levels of stress affect pregnenolone and causes hormonal imbalance in oestrogen, progesterone, causing them to deplete faster and leads to a quicker and painful menopause.

5. Have spiritual grounding (need not be religious).

6. Engage in yoga under supervision.

7. Divert your mind.

8. Change your environment.

9. Start with guided meditation.

10. Serotonin-boosting food: Avocado, grapes, shitake mushrooms (rich in B6 precursor of serotonin), sesame seeds (precursor of tyrosine that increases brain dopamine levels), strawberries serve as a strong line of defence against brain degeneration, also boosting happy chemicals.

- Vaginal dryness and decreased sex drive

Due to menopause, there is a reduction in oestrogen hormones, the vaginal lining becomes thin and that is why dryness sets in.

Vaginal dryness during intercourse might be painful and unsatisfying.

Solution:

For Dryness:

1. Apply 99 per cent pure aloe vera gel in the vaginal area.

2. Mix 1 tbsp cold pressed coconut oil (anti-bacterial) with a pinch of organic turmeric powder (anti-inflammatory).

3. Take a bucket of water, add 1 tbsp apple cider vinegar (ACV) with mother, immerse groin area for 15–20

minutes (in case of cuts, avoid ACV as it may lead to a burning sensation). In case of cuts in vaginal area due to dryness, you can take warm water with ½ tsp organic turmeric powder and immerse your groin area for 15–20 minutes.

4. Break vitamin E capsules and apply in vaginal area.

- Libido

  1. Unroasted 1 tsp flax seeds and walnuts.

  2. Zinc-rich food: Soak 1–2 tsp pumpkin seeds.

  3. Libido-boosting concoction: ½ tsp methi seeds, a pinch of nutmeg, saffron, 1 clove garlic; boil for 15 minutes, strain and add honey; consume 1 hour before bedtime.

  4. Involve in foreplay for 15–20 minutes.

  5. Consume dry dates 1 hour before bedtime with pistachios.

  6. Add jasmine essential oil to a diffuser since it helps uplift your mood.

- Increased abdominal fat and weight gain

Solution:

1. Let's not look at this from a vanity or numerical viewpoint. You should work towards reducing your fat per cent. The weighing scale is not a benchmark, but let's work on inch loss.

2. Be physically active. 10,000 steps is a must. In case you have any physical ailments, check with your doctor before settling on a goal. Probiotics are healthy bacteria that can actually improve your production and regulation of key hormones like insulin, ghrelin and leptin, which manage food intake. The best sources include yoghurt, kefir,

cultured veggies such as sauerkraut or kimchi, kombucha and other fermented food like idli, dosa, etc.

3. Add a good amount of fibre along with other nutrients.

4. 1 glass water with a pinch of Sri Lankan rolled cinnamon powder.

5. Add a cup of green tea/matcha tea.

6. Add a dash of cayenne pepper to gravies.

- Insomnia and changes in sleep quality

Solution:

1. Keep the room dark and cooler.

2. Warm water bath 30 minutes before bedtime, add 1–2 drops of valerian root essential oil, it will help you calm down.

3. Warm water bath with Epsom salt works well too due to its magnesium content.

4. Listen to yoga nidra/InsightTimer App.

5. Add a pinch of nutmeg powder to a cup of water at bedtime.

6. Sip on camomile tea towards the evening.

7. Do not sleep during the day, rest well at night.

- Thinning hair and dry skin

Solution:

1. Mask: Half avocado and half a banana; apply the mask on scalp for 30 minutes and then wash.

2. 1 tsp soaked (overnight) methi seeds mixed with A2 curd.

3. Apply pure aloe vera gel.

4. 500 ml mustard oil, 200 ml coconut oil, 1 tsp curry leaf powder, 1 tbsp methi seeds; infuse for 1 week and apply.

5. Apply cold pressed coconut oil on skin or 99 per cent pure aloe vera gel.

- Going to the bathroom more often

Solution:

1. Check if you are on any diuretics.

2. Caffeine and alcohol also increases frequent washroom visits. Try and limit or avoid caffeine.

3. Practice Kegel exercises.

- Breast changes (including breasts becoming smaller or losing volume)

Solution:

1. Take 2 tsp olive oil and rub it between your palms. Massage it gently on your breasts for 5–10 minutes. Do this once or twice daily.

2. Pour warm and cold water alternatively on your breasts to release skin proteins responsible for skin tone and tightening, and enhance the blood flow to the skin.

- Changes in the uterus, ovaries and cervix

Solution:

1. One can engage in yoga in the premenopausal stage that will involve a good massage for abdominal organs.

2. Kapalbhati, anulom vilom and pranayama help, too.

Note: Practice under supervision.

Besides the above, there are a lot of changes happening during menopause that can be managed well.

These are listed below:

1. Cognition/memory is affected; hence, add memory-boosting food like: cacao, rosemary oil, avocados, blueberries, broccoli, celery, cold pressed coconut oil, beetroot, bone broth, egg yolk (due to choline), almonds, salmon, turmeric, walnuts and brahmi.

2. Playing chess, board games, solving puzzles and crosswords will help boost brain health.

3. Studies show that excessive stress and poor sleep are linked with higher levels of cortisol, decreased immunity, trouble with work performance, and a higher susceptibility to anxiety, weight gain and depression. To allow your body to recover from stress, control your appetite and improve your energy, aim to get 7–9 hours of sleep every night.

4. Gamma-aminobutyric acids (GABA) act as neurotransmitters in your brain. Fermented foods rich in probiotics (fermented pickles, sauerkraut, kimchi, kefir, etc.) help to increase GABA levels.

5. Walking, running, jogging, swimming and cycling are some exercises that can keep the nervous system healthy.

6. Sudoku, brain teasers, puzzles and aptitude tests can help improve motor skills. Simple tasks like doing calculations without a calculator can also keep your mind sharp.

7. If you are acidic, your body leaches calcium from your bones to make the system alkaline, hence reducing bone density. Besides, during menopause, oestrogen, the hormone that protects bones during fertile periods, is lacking, posing a further threat to calcium de-mineralization. It's important to work on acidity by adding alkaline foods like cucumber,

lemon water, aloe vera juice, etc. to your diet. A simple hack to combat acidity is to suck a clove or cardamom. Keep your D3 level in check.

A Few Factors to Take into Consideration besides Managing Menopausal Symptoms Include:

1. Organic fruits and vegetables contain dietary fibre to manage your appetite, antioxidants to slow the ageing process, and phytosterols that can help balance hormones.

2. Fibre is important for cardiovascular and digestive health, plus maintaining healthy weight. Some studies have even found that diets higher in fibre might help balance production of oestrogen. Some of the best sources include nuts, seeds, legumes/beans, ancient grains, avocados, vegetables and fruit.

3. Fermented soy like natto contains a phytoestrogen that can help balance hormones. However, avoid this if you have had oestrogen-positive breast cancer in the past. If you are adding this product, ensure it is not produced using GMOs and take it in moderation.

4. Unrefined oils are also the building blocks for hormone production; they keep inflammation levels low, boost your metabolism, and promote satiety that is important for preventing weight gain. Unrefined oils provide essential vitamin E that helps regulate oestrogen production. Look for virgin coconut oil, sesame oil, mustard oil, groundnut oil. Other sources of healthy fats include avocado, coconut milk, nuts, seeds, etc.

5. Aim for 10–12 glasses daily to help replace fluid lost from hot flashes and to decrease bloating.

6. As an adaptogenic herb, maca has been used for thousands of years to lower the effects of stress and ageing on the body by decreasing cortisol levels. It can

help with hot flashes, low energy/fatigue, restlessness and weight gain while improving libido and energy.

7. Adaptogens include ashwagandha, medicinal mushrooms, rhodiola, liquorice and holy basil. Research shows they can help improve thyroid function, lower cholesterol, reduce anxiety and depression, reduce brain cell degeneration, and stabilize blood sugar and insulin levels. (We can opt for 1 each month before moving to the next.)

8. Clary sage oil is the most effective essential oil for balancing hormones. It can help offer relief from menopause symptoms including increased anxiety and hot flashes. In addition, camomile oil reduces stress, peppermint oil can help cool the body from hot flashes, and thyme oil can help naturally balance hormones. You can rub 3 drops of the chosen oil on the tops of your feet, and the back of your neck 1–3 times daily. You can combine any essential oil with a carrier oil like jojoba or coconut oil to dilute its strength and decrease skin sensitivity.

9. Cooked banana flower eaten with A2 curd is effective for menstrual disorders like excessive bleeding, and painful menstruation.

10. Ginger, turmeric, fennel, anise, sage and blackseed are a few spices to consume during pre-menopause to ease the menopausal symptoms.

11. Optimal B12 levels are important to reduce depression and for healthy nerve health.

12. Avoid packaged food, conventional meat, sugar, refined oil and fried products, carbonated beverages, and alcohol.

Hacks to Take Care of Oral Hygiene

1. Use a neem twig to brush.

2. Chew on some bamboo sticks.
3. Rinse your mouth after every meal.
4. Oil pulling.

Here is a DIY mouthwash recipe:

Ingredients:

- 2 cups water
- 2 tbsp cold pressed coconut oil
- 1 tsp (heaped) pink Himalayan salt/rock salt
- 3–4 drops of peppermint essential oil

Method:

1. Mix ingredients in a glass container and shake well until salt dissolves.
2. Use as much as required. You'll have to shake the container before each use.
3. If the coconut oil solidifies, you can run the glass jar under warm water.

Note:

When using, swish and gargle around a mouthful of the mixture for 30 seconds before spitting it out. Use in the morning or whenever you feel that your mouth is stale during the day.

Home Remedies for Diaper Dermatitis

1. Expose the baby's bottom to air for some time during the day to keep diaper rash from settling in.
2. Coconut oil is among the foremost natural products that will work wonders especially for diaper dermatitis caused by yeast. Studies indicate that copra oil is anti-fungal, especially against candida albicans, a kind of fungus.

3. You can also cure diaper rash by applying topical barriers to the diaper region like petrolatum or petroleum jelly.

4. If your baby's diaper rash causes severe inflammation, then you ought to use aloe vera gel.

5. Cornstarch is extremely good for treating rashes because it helps to scale back diaper friction. After removing the soiled diaper, wash your baby's bottom with lukewarm water and dry the skin carefully with a soft cloth. Lightly sprinkle cornstarch on the skin directly a bit like powder before using a new diaper. Repeat till the skin heals completely.

6. Dilute 1 tsp of apple cider vinegar in a cup of water and wash your baby's bottom at the time of adjusting the diaper.

7. Breast milk has many amazing bio-dynamic properties; it often is a safe, effective and convenient remedy for soothing diaper dermatitis. Simply apply a few drops of breast milk on the rash-affected area at regular intervals and let it dry naturally.

8. Plain yoghurt is good for diaper rashes and inflammation.

9. Oatmeal bath is a tried and tested remedy for diaper dermatitis in babies. It provides relief from the pain. Grind ⅓ cup of oats to form a fine powder; then mix this powder slowly into lukewarm bathwater. Hold your baby in a sitting position in the bathtub and for 10–15 minutes, then pat his skin dry (do not rub).

10. Mix 2 tbsp of baking soda in lukewarm water and wash the rash-affected area with this solution at regular intervals. Don't wipe, let it dry naturally.

Home Remedies for Baby Colic

1. Feeding: Breastfeeding is best for infants. Feed your

baby in smaller quantities at frequent intervals of 1½ to 2 hours by keeping him/her as upright as possible. Then make your baby burp by gently patting on the rear after each feed. If you're feeding formula milk to your infant, try another brand; babies can sometimes be sensitive to certain brands of protein in formula milk. Moreover, the mother's diet also matters; a hypoallergenic diet may cause colic pain. Breastfeeding mothers should avoid tea, coffee, spicy food and alcohol.

2. Cuddling: Cuddling is among the foremost effective remedies for colic. Babies respond to skin to skin contact; when you hold your baby close, she feels secure and the crying subsides. By rocking your baby gently in your arms, you can also make your baby sleep peacefully.

3. Create a noise: Noises can often refocus a baby's attention, and reduce crying overall. For instance, recreate the noise of a fan, washer, vacuum cleaner, etc. It'll help appease your baby.

4. Warm compress: A lukewarm compress on your baby's tummy will provide some relief since colic is typically caused by problems within the gastrointestinal system. A warm towel on the stomach will work as well.

5. Use of probiotics: Probiotics help increase good bacteria, enhance intestinal function and aid in digestion of food. Rice kanji can also be a solution.

6. Massage with oil: Massaging with mustard, coconut or sesame oil can help to subside a baby's crying; it'll make the baby feel relaxed and calm by improving blood circulation.

7. Asafoetida: Asafoetida is also good for alleviating baby colic pain. Take a solid block, break a pinch of asafoetida and make a paste by adding a small

amount of warm water. Apply this paste over the navel area of the baby; it helps release gas from the stomach.

Home Remedies for Deworming

1. Ajwain with Jaggery:
   a) Simply grind some carom seeds to form a fine powder and blend thoroughly with some jaggery. Make small balls (1–2 gm each) from this mixture. Now, ingest 1 ball with water.
   b) Ajwain with buttermilk: After grinding carom seeds, add ½ gm powder to buttermilk.

2. Ripe tomato for deworming: Give 1–2 tomatoes with a pinch of rock salt and black pepper to your child to eat on an empty stomach for a few days; it kills stomach worms. Please make sure that he shouldn't eat anything for up to 2 hours after eating tomatoes.

3. Radish juice: 10 ml radish juice is an effective deworming treatment.

4. Curd: Curd removes intestinal parasites naturally through excretion without any additional medication.

5. Amla juice: Grate or grind 2–3 amlas and extract the juice with the assistance of a thin cloth. 5 gm of fresh amla juice with some honey on an empty stomach works wonders for deworming.

6. Neem leaves: Grind one cup of tender neem leaves. Add carom seeds and black salt with a pinch of dry ginger powder to the neem leaves paste. After mixing well, make small balls (1 gm each) of this paste and dry completely in sunlight.

7. Garlic: Garlic contains allicin, an oily liquid with antibacterial properties. Consume raw garlic on an empty stomach for best results.

8. Coconut: Coconut has very strong anti-parasitic properties. Give your child a small piece of coconut to eat on an empty stomach for a week.

9. Carrot: Carrot is not only used to treat threadworms, but also for deworming of other parasites.

10. Tulsi leaves: First, crush 15–20 basil leaves after washing thoroughly. Extract the juice with a sieve by pressing with fingertips. Now, give 1 tsp of basil juice to your child for deworming.

11. Papaya leaves: Papaya can help destroy intestinal worms. Put 200 ml of water in a pan along with the leaves and boil this water till it reduces in half. Let it cool, then mix with honey before drinking.

12. Unripe papaya: For deworming, take 3–5 tbsp extract of unripe papaya and 1 tbsp of honey.

13. Turmeric: Turmeric or haldi is/may be a natural antiseptic and antibacterial spice. Mix ¼–1 tsp in lukewarm water and provide it to your child on an empty stomach.

14. Onion juice: Give 1–2 spoons of onion juice to your kid with honey on an empty stomach.

15. Drumstick seeds: By consuming two grams of drumstick seed powder with water, intestinal worms are going to be killed and removed.

16. Bitter gourd juice: Bitter gourd juice helps to clear intestinal worms. Since the juice is bitter, add a little honey for your little one.

17. Banana with lemon juice: Mash a bit of ripe banana and blend with 1 tsp of juice.

18. Pomegranate juice: 30–40 ml pomegranate (anar) juice is good for deworming.

19. Pumpkin seeds: Pumpkin seeds contain a compound, cucurbitacin, and a few other worm-killing properties

that help paralyse the worms within the body and stop their growth. Therefore, eat 8–10 pumpkin seeds daily for 7–8 days to kill intestinal worms.

20. Giloy: ½ tsp giloy with honey works well.

Natural Remedies for Cold among Kids

1. Ginger and basil juice: Ginger and basil plants have mucus-releasing properties. Mix 4–5 drops of ginger juice and 4–5 drops of basil juice for best results.

2. Alum: Alum's natural antimicrobial properties could cure cold and cough among kids. First, take some alum and grind into a fine powder. Roast over a low flame until it melts. Let it cool and grind again to form a fine powder. Keep this powder in an airtight jar and use when required. Give a pinch (½–1 gm) of this powder to your child with honey to cure cough.

3. Figs: Soak a dry fig in some water. Blend and give this paste to your child.

4. Carom seeds: Carom seeds and dry ginger are best for curing cold and cough. Lightly roast carom seeds on a pan for 2–3 minutes and grind into a powder. Grind some dry ginger to form a fine powder. Mix carom seed powder and dry ginger powder (1 gm each) in 1 tsp of honey.

5. Flax seed decoction: Flax seed decoction may be a highly effective home remedy for curing a child's chronic cold. Boil 1 tsp of flax seeds in 200 ml water for ten minutes. Strain the decoction into a cup and mix 2 tbsp of water before giving it to your child.

6. Carom seed compress: Take some carom seeds and make a poultice with soft cotton. Place the poultice on a pre-heated pan and dab it when lukewarm on the chest, back, palms and soles of your baby.

7. Chebulic myrobalan: Grind some harad (terminalia chebula) after lightly roasting on a pan. Keep it in a jar after making a fine powder. Give a pinch or two of this powder with honey to young children, twice a day.

Home Remedies for Cradle Cap

1. Coconut oil: Coconut oil's anti-fungal and antibacterial properties make it a good choice to treat cradle cap. Gently apply a few drops of copra oil on the scalp. Leave it for 15–20 minutes. Olive oil can be used, too. It is good for the skin because it contains vitamin E.

2. Petrolatum: It helps maintain skin moisture; it also helps remove greasy patches on a toddler's scalp caused by dermatitis. Apply petrolatum on your baby's scalp in the dark and leave it overnight. Wash the hair with mild baby shampoo in the morning and wipe with a soft towel.

3. Bicarbonate of soda: It helps absorb excess oil that clogs the pores. Therefore, mix a few spoons of baking soda with equal amount of water, apply over the scalp and leave it for 5–7 minutes.

4. Breast milk: Apply a few drops of breast milk on the affected area of the scalp and leave it for some time; then brush gently.

5. Almond oil: Almond oil is rich in vitamin E and works against dermatitis, too. Apply it on the affected area of the scalp of the baby and massage gently.

6. Baby hair brush: Brush your baby's scalp with a soft baby hair brush at least twice a day. It helps remove greasy patches and maintain hygiene, too. Don't apply force; it'll take time to cure completely.

Luke's Khichdi Corner

Khichdi is widely prepared in many Indian states such as Haryana, Rajasthan, Gujarat, West Bengal, Assam, Bihar, Jharkhand, Uttar Pradesh and Maharashtra. An elaborate yet easy recipe, khichdi makes for a wholesome yet delicious meal. It can be made with a variety of ingredients, not just whole spices, but also onions, garlic and tomatoes. In many Indian households, it is one of the first solid foods that babies eat. If you don't have time to prepare a kadhi, you can just serve it with curd and you have a sumptuous dinner on the table!

Khichdi for Senior Citizens

Ingredients:

- 1 cup hand pounded *sona masuri* rice
- 1 cup split green moong dal
- 3 tsp ghee
- 1 tsp cumin
- 1 bay leaf
- ½ tsp asafoetida
- ½ tsp turmeric powder
- Coriander leaves (to garnish)

Method:

1. In a pressure cooker, add ghee followed by cumin and bay leaves.

2. Add the soaked rice and dal.

3. Add salt, turmeric and hing.

4. Add water and cook for 4–5 whistles until all the ingredients are combined well.

5. Served hot with a dollop of ghee.

Variations:

Khichdi can be relished by children and senior citizens too.

Adding bottle gourd, sweet potato or pumpkin to the khichdi not only adds to the nutrient value but gives it extra taste as well, and it is the best way to introduce these vegetables to fussy eaters.

Masala Khichdi

Ingredients:

- 1 cup rice (parboiled, soaked for 8 hours)
- ½ cup moong dal/green gram split (pre-soaked for 8–10 hours)
- ¾ cup toor dal (pre-soaked for 8–10 hours)
- ¼ cup urad dal (pre-soaked for 8–10 hours)
- 2 tbsp finely chopped moringa leaves
- 5–6 cups water
- 1 finely chopped onion
- 1 finely chopped tomato
- 1 cup mix of pumpkin, carrots, beans and fresh peas/mushrooms
- 2 tsp grated ginger
- 4–5 chopped garlic cloves
- 1 star anise
- 1 tsp mustard seeds 1 tbsp secret masala
- ½ tsp red chilli powder

- 1 tbsp ghee
- Pink salt to taste
- Coriander leaves (to garnish)

Method:

1. Wash rice and dal, drain and keep aside.

2. Heat ghee in pressure cooker pan, add the star anise and mustard seeds, and allow them to splutter. Add ginger, garlic and onion.

3. Sauté till onion turns pink.

4. Add tomatoes. Once the oil begins to separate, add garam masala, red chilli powder, vegetable mix and moringa.

5. Now add water.

6. Once the water starts boiling, add rice and dal.

7. Cover and pressure cook (4–5 whistles).

8. Serve hot with ghee.

9. Garnish with fresh coriander leaves.

Jain Khichdi

Ingredients:

- 1 cup hand-pounded sona masuri rice
- ½ cup green moong dal
- ¼ cup black urad dal
- ¼ cup masoor dal
- ½ cup mixed vegetables (bottle gourd, peas and cabbage)
- ¼ cup chopped tomatoes
- 1 tsp cumin
- ¼ tsp pepper
- ¼ tsp immunity powder

- 1 inch grated ginger
- A pinch of asafoetida
- 4–5 curry leaves
- 2 tbsp ghee
- Salt
- 4–5 cups water

Method:

1. Wash the pre-soaked dals and rice and pressure cook with 4–5 cups water until 5 whistles.

2. Set aside.

3. Heat 2 tbsp A2 ghee in a pan, add pepper, cumin seeds, grated ginger, immunity powder, curry leaves and asafoetida and sauté.

4. Now add the chopped tomatoes and mixed vegetables. Cover and cook well.

5. Pour the tomato and mixed vegetables over the rice mixture and stir.

6. Serve hot with a dollop of ghee.

Indian Food: A Combination of Good Protein

I want to talk about protein and link it back to one of our staple meals in India, the humble dal chawal or rice and dal. There's this whole myth about protein and how much you need, but what's more important is the quality of protein that you consume every day. The media and the market have us believing that consumption of protein and lean muscle build-up is directly proportional, that the bigger we get, the more muscle we have. A lot of women believe that increasing protein intake reduces fat content in the body. That does make a little bit of sense, because if you have a good amount of protein in your body you can build lean mass but it doesn't always have to be quantity over quality. It is always quality over quantity because it doesn't matter how much protein you have. What really matters is how this protein breaks down into amino acids in your body. So, for example, you may get 30 grams of protein in a scoop of any whey protein that you spend about Rs 3500–4000 a month, and you may have a tablespoon of pumpkin seeds that contains 3–4 grams of protein, but quality protein with all the amino acids is the perfect combination.

Having the right amount of protein in your diet is extremely beneficial. Not only does it make you look good and give you that muscle tone, but the more muscle tone you have, the higher your metabolic activity and it's all about metabolism. The higher your metabolism, the faster you lose weight.

So overtraining, under-eating and starvation diets will help you make temporary gains until you put on weight again because you ignored your metabolic activity. Weight loss is not about just exercise and diet; it's about communication between your hormones. Are you giving your body the right energy it needs?

Your cells require energy so that your immunity can fight viruses, pathogens and germs. Your white blood cells break down lean mass and that's protein, because it uses protein to heal itself. Protein is the building block of cells. This means cells are constantly dying and growing all the time. It needs energy. It needs protein. But it needs quality protein.

Our staple Indian dal and rice is one of the best combinations and one of the most complete proteins. What do I mean by a complete protein? There are twenty amino acids. Nine of them are essential. Our body cannot manufacture these nine amino acids which means we need to consume food items rich in these amino acids.

For example, lentils have an amino acid called lysine that rice does not have and rice has all the sulphur-based amino acids absent in lentils.

Visit a village and you'll see men and women with strong,

lean bodies. Their physical activity is at a higher level than us city dwellers and their staple diet is lentils, grains and vegetables. They don't have protein shakes or supplements or any of the things we think we need to achieve a lean body, and yet they're so lean and ripped eating carbohydrates, lentils and everything that we're scared of.

So yes, you should have that dal chawal in your diet. Now, what's important is variety. Our country is blessed with a variety of lentils and legumes. From rajmas and chanas to our green, yellow and orange dals, we have it all. Look for variety because one dal may contain the essential nutrients missing from a different variety. So your simple dal chawal happens to be very nutritious food. It won't be the same as a scoop of whey protein, but we need to keep things simple. We have to go back to our roots and understand it's about a complete protein, a quality protein, and not just the quantity of protein.

Food Synergy

Certain foods complement each other so well that they seem to make each other better! As though they were meant to be together, they blend with each other in a synergistic rhythm. I call such food pairings—'The Perfect Food Couples'.

What if I told you that certain food combinations not only amp up the flavour but improve their overall nutritional value? Certain ingredients, when used together, turn them from individually regular dishes into healing superfoods. Certain combinations can help provide better nourishment by improving the body's ability to utilize these nutrients, also called bioavailability.

This concept of 'food synergy' may be nature's own meal plan to make us fitter. Try combining some of these synergistic foods in your diet for a healthier you:

1. Lemon and Green Tea

   Squirt some lemon juice into your morning cuppa. The vitamin C in the lemon facilitates the absorption of the green tea's antioxidants—catechins—in the body.

   Caffeine-containing beverages such as green tea tend to make our body acidic.

   Lemon helps to make the body pH alkaline and hence, adding lemon juice to the green tea will help to buffer acidity.

2. Fish and Garlic

   Garlic has sulphur compounds that help boost one's immunity and also reduce bad cholesterol levels. Fish being rich in protein and omega-3 also boosts one's immunity and reduces inflammation in the body. Use garlic in your fish marinade to help boost the therapeutic properties of fish and garlic and to drop the LDL and triglyceride levels. This combination of foods does the job more efficiently together than when eaten separately.

3. Rosemary and Steak

   The robust flavour of rosemary goes very well with a meat steak. Using rosemary to marinate or flavour your steak helps neutralize the carcinogenic compounds such as heterocyclic amine (HCA) that are formed when you char the meat or cook it at a high temperature. This is due to the high antioxidant content such as carnosic acid and carnosol in rosemary. Always make sure you consume grass-fed, organic meat.

4. Vinegar and Rice

   Vinegar helps improve insulin sensitivity. Combining vinegar with a rice-based meal helps to shallow out and prevent spikes in blood sugar levels by 20–35 per cent. This is particularly important for someone who is diabetic or simply watching their weight.

5. Tomato and Olive Oil

   Tomatoes are rich in phytochemicals called lycopene that help fight prostate cancer by improving prostate health and prevent heart disease. These carotenoids are fat-soluble; thus drizzling a little olive oil on tomatoes makes them easily available to the body.

6. Lemon and Spinach

   Spinach has an abundance of iron. Being a plant-based (non-heme) source of iron, the bioavailability of this nutrient in the body is poor. Vitamin C in lemon helps improve absorption of iron into the body.

Vitamin C aids in better absorption of iron from all iron-containing plant-based sources such as garden cress seeds and wheatgrass. Simply add soaked garden cress seeds or wheatgrass powder to a glass of water with some lemon juice mixed to help that iron turn bioavailable.

7. Turmeric and Pepper

We've all heard of the numerous benefits of haldi, ranging from healing wounds to reducing the sniffles. Turmeric also has a lot of benefits such as boosting immunity, lowering cholesterol, improving liver function, etc. However, curcumin (the active component of turmeric) is not absorbed and passes through our system only to be flushed out mostly unused. Consuming pepper with turmeric increases the absorption of curcumin multifold by making it bio-available to us.

One must look for curcumin along with piperine when buying a curcumin supplement. If you don't have piperine added in the supplement, it is important to add a pinch of pepper to the water while swallowing the pill for better bioavailability.

8. Vitamin E and Selenium

On their own, selenium and vitamin E are superfoods for boosting immunity and reducing gut and skin issues. However, combining the two nutrients seems to have a better effect on reducing inflammation. Studies have shown a decrease in proliferation markers of prostate cancer when treated with a combination of vitamin E and selenium.

- A few sources of vitamin E are almonds, peanuts, hazelnuts, sunflower seeds, green leafy vegetables like spinach, broccoli and wheatgerm.

- Sources of selenium include Brazil nuts, fish, whole grain cereals, chicken, eggs, mushrooms, lentils, banana, brown rice and oatmeal.

To get the best out of both, you could have some grilled fish with steamed broccoli on the side; sprinkle your oatmeal with lightly roasted almonds and sunflower seeds; or combine the spinach with mushroom to enjoy these sautéed veggies with steamed brown rice. Experiment away and make your own combination.

9. Calcium and Vitamin D

Vitamin D facilitates the absorption of calcium in the body. When vitamin D levels are low, no matter how much calcium you pump into your system, it won't be absorbed. This is the reason why your calcium supplement will also have a small amount of vitamin D.

Very few foods in nature contain vitamin D, although a few sources include fatty fish (salmon, tuna, mackerel), egg yolks, and mushrooms are rich in it.

Combining these foods with calcium-rich food sources such as broccoli, cabbage, non-GMO soya bean, seeds (sesame, poppy, chia, almonds, etc.), beans and dairy products will help improve overall nutritional intake.

Whole eggs with a glass of A2 organic cow milk make for a perfect breakfast and it's great for healthy bones. Egg yolks, rich in vitamin D, increase the absorption of calcium from milk. This is particularly important to prevent brittle bones and osteoporosis.

In case of lactose intolerance, you can opt for a nut-based milk like almond milk with the egg for your calcium needs; or else add chopped spinach to your egg omelette.

We must also appreciate the power of magnesium and

its importance in allowing calcium do its job. It has now been established that magnesium is the key to the body's proper assimilation and use of calcium.

Magnesium is found in whole grains, cacao, nuts, seafood, legumes, peas, carrots and green leafy vegetables. Having said that, too much calcium without adequately balancing it with magnesium may cause a magnesium deficiency or malabsorption and can have adverse effects on the body. The body tends to either store or recycle calcium. Magnesium, on the other hand, is either used up or excreted from our body and needs to be replenished on a regular basis.

10. Cereals and Pulses

Our Indian diet is traditionally plant-based with a majority of the population being vegetarian or lacto-vegetarian, and consumption of meat is fairly low. A conventional Indian thali is a well-balanced combination of lentils with rotis or dal and rice or khichdi which is an ideal cereal and pulse combination.

This combination in the right ratio enables us to get the required amount of complete protein that is otherwise lacking in a vegetarian diet.

We need complete protein to boost our immunity, for repair and recovery of cells, and muscle building.

This beautiful synergy of ingredients, which is an intrinsic part of our native culture, is what we need to keep in mind to stay healthy and receive maximum nourishment from everything we eat.

Good food is made great when eaten intelligently. By understanding how our incredibly complex bodies work, we can adjust our diets to best suit it and aid it along the way to wellness and good health.

Disclaimer: We do not promote these food combinations as a replacement/substitute for any medication/treatment/ supplement. Please consult your nutritionist, doctor and other healthcare professionals regarding supplement recommendations or medical advice or before trying anything new or trying a remedy/superfood/hack as per your individual requirements/ capacity and health conditions/issues/discomfort.

Recipes

Fermented Beverages

Not only do beverages provide essential hydration but they can also be a source of other nutrients. Besides energy, some beverages are a source of vitamins, minerals, protein, fats and other carbohydrates.

1. Raabdi
2. Carrot/Beetroot Kanji

Raabdi

Raabdi is a regular drink popular across the rural regions of Rajasthan. The beverage is made by using curd or buttermilk and barley flour. It is served hot with regular dinner during winters. One can also use jowar instead of barley.

Ingredients:

- 2 tbsp roasted barley flour
- 1½ cup buttermilk
- Cumin (for garnishing)
- Salt to taste

Method:

1. Mix buttermilk and barley flour in a bowl and add salt

to it. Mix well so no lumps are left in the liquid.

2. Cover it with a lid and keep it aside for 1–2 hours. (Traditionally it is made and kept in the sun for natural fermentation in an earthen pot.)

3. Pour it into a saucepan and cook it on a low flame stirring continuously, preferably with a wooden ladle, for about 25–30 minutes. You will notice it thickens while cooking.

4. Stop cooking when it reaches a semi-liquid consistency.

5. Sprinkle raw cumin seeds to garnish. Raab/raabdi will thicken further upon cooling.

Notes:

- Cooking increases the number of antioxidants.
- A study reveals that on fermentation, the amount of protein increases in pearl millet (12.2 per cent–20.3 per cent)
- Another study revealed that when fermentation was carried out in an earthen pot, there was an increase in the amount of antioxidants or quercetins.
- It has a cooling effect on the digestive tract.
- The presence of buttermilk provides probiotics, phosphorus and calcium.
- It encourages digestion by promoting good bacteria.
- It helps boost the immune system.
- Barley is high in fibre and curbs hunger, thus helping in weight reduction.

Nutrition Table:

Calories (kcal)	Carbohydrates (g)	Protein (g)	Fat (g)
100	14	3.8	3.2

Carrot/Beetroot Kanji

Kanji, a self-fermented beverage, is used as a traditional medicine in several Asian countries to treat gastrointestinal and liver disorders, and increase appetite. Preparing kanji includes the use of naturally-occurring bacteria in the air and yeast present in vegetable skin. This is why, it may be best not to peel the carrots.

Ingredients:

- 1 cup carrots, unpeeled, cut into 1 inch sticks
- 1 cup beetroot, unpeeled, cut into 1 inch sticks
- 2 tbsp ground mustard powder
- ½ tsp Kashmiri chilli powder
- 4–5 cups of water

Method:

Put all the ingredients into a big glass jar. Screw on the lid and leave in a warm corner to ferment for at least 3 days. You can also leave it in the sun till it ferments. Fermentation might take longer in winter. It has a sour, pungent taste.

Serves 4–5

Notes:

- Drink about half a cup first thing each morning to awaken your body, mind and spirit to another glorious day.
- Fermented food has the unique ability to ease digestive discomfort related to having either too much or too little stomach acid. When the production of hydrochloric acid by the stomach is low, fermented food helps increase the acidity of gastric juices. On the other hand, when the stomach produces too much acid, fermented food helps protect the stomach and intestinal lining.

Accompaniments

Accompaniments are complementary additions to the main ingredient of a meal. They typically comprise chutney powder, pickles and chutneys. It's used to bring balance to an array of dishes, highlight a specific flavour profile, and also add an anti-inflammatory quality to the plate.

1. Kollu Podi
2. Kuzhambu
3. Menthe (Menthyada) Hittu/Methkoot
4. Gobi Gajar Shalgam Achaar
5. Luke's Immunity-Boosting Powder and Chutney

Kollu Podi

Ingredients:

- 1 cup horse gram
- 5 red chillies
- ¼ tsp asafoetida
- 3 garlic cloves
- 1 sprig of curry leaves
- 1 tsp salt
- 1 tsp sesame oil/cooking oil

Method:

1. Heat 1 tsp oil in a pan and roast the horse gram, curry leaves, garlic cloves, red chilli and asafoetida together on a low flame for a minimum of 5 minutes. Keep stirring.
2. Transfer it to a plate and let it cool down.
3. Now transfer all these roasted ingredients with salt into your food processor and coarsely grind them. Store it in a dry, airtight container.

Notes:

Horse gram is a low profile legume but is rich in calcium, iron and proteins. My grandma used to make Kollu Podi in winters as it has the power to energize your system and provide warmth. We usually mix this horse gram powder with steamed rice, drizzle some sesame oil or ghee, and enjoy. You can use this powder as a dry chutney too, like palli podi or idli.

Kuzhumbu

Kuzhumbu is a cleansing food. There are no vegetables involved, no onion or garlic, and no extra spices. A very simple south Indian style pachadi (similar to a yoghurt-based raita with a tadka) and a papad (preferably sutta appalam) are served as side dishes. Kuzhumbu is a very common recipe in the Tamil Brahmin community. Kuzhumbu along with kootu (vegetable and moong dal-based gravy) is believed to be a medicinal food, light for the tummy, and is great for nursing mothers. During rainy days or when you have a severe cold and cough, this simple curry is the best medicine.

Ingredients:

To roast and grind:
- 2 tbsp urad dal
- 2 tbsp toor dal
- 2 tbsp black peppercorns
- 1 dry red chilli
- ½ tsp coriander seeds

For curry:
- ½ tsp mustard seeds
- ½ tsp cumin
- 2 cups tamarind extract

- ¼ cup curry leaves
- ½ tbsp salt
- ½ tbsp jaggery (optional)

Method:

1. Soak lemon-sized tamarind in warm water for 20 minutes.
2. Extract tamarind water and filter out the impurities.
3. Heat some oil in a non-stick frying pan.
4. Add urad dal and toor dal and sauté until they are golden brown.
5. Add chilli, black peppercorns, coriander seeds and continue sautéing for 3–4 minutes.
6. After it cools, grind the mixture into a coarse powder.
7. In the same pan, add oil, mustard seeds, cumin seeds and curry leaves.
8. Let them splutter.
9. Add tamarind water, salt, hing and turmeric.
10. Let the mixture boil on low flame for 5 minutes.
11. Add the ground (pepper and dal) powder and stir well.
12. Let the mixture boil on a low flame for 10–12 minutes.
13. The curry will start to thicken. If you are adding jaggery, stir it in now. Curry is ready.

Notes:

- Very flavourful.
- Tamarind and dal add to the flavour.

Menthe (Menthyada) Hittu/Methkoot

This dish is popular in north Karnataka and Maharashtra. Made from various mixed pulses and grains, Methkoot is rich in protein, nutritious and delicious. Mix it with some hot rice, top it with a little ghee and relish.

Ingredients:

- 1 cup white urad dal (whole)
- 1 cup chana dal
- 1 cup arhar dal (split dal)
- ½ cup yellow moong dal (split)
- 2–3 tsp horse gram
- 2 tsp rice
- 4–5 tsp broken jowar
- 1 tsp fenugreek seeds
- 2–3 tsp coriander seeds
- 2 tsp cumin seeds
- ¼ tsp whole black peppercorns
- 4 dry red chillies
- ½ cup curry leaves
- 1 tsp turmeric powder
- ½ tsp asafoetida

Method:

1. In a frying pan, dry-roast each ingredient separately on a medium-low flame till they are crisp and aromatic.
2. Take care not to burn anything.
3. Let all the ingredients cool to room temperature. Grind them to a very smooth powder along with some salt in a grinder.
4. Store it in an airtight container.

Notes:

- The menthe hittu chutney powder can be served with plain hot rice and also goes well with chapatis or dosas.
- Use as topping on bhel, upma or on any chat preparation.
- Use in vegetarian or non-vegetarian frankie as masala.
- Use in side dishes like koshimbir and salads.
- Use it to make curries flavourful and thick
- Use it as a rub on your favourite meat.
- Use it as a coating for spiced nuts.
- Methkoot is low in calories and high in iron and folate, and is an excellent source of protein and dietary fibre.
- It helps prevent constipation and other digestive disorders like IBS.
- It is an excellent source of protein for vegetarians and vegans.
- Dietary fibre helps to reduce blood cholesterol levels and lowers the risk of heart disease.
- Magnesium is a mineral used in building bones and muscles.
- It helps boost metabolism and helps keep blood vessels healthy.
- It has antioxidant properties that ease inflammation.

Gajar Gobhi Shalgam ka Achaar

Ingredients:

- 500 gm carrots cut into 1½ inch pieces
- 500 gm cauliflower separated into florets
- 500 gm turnips peeled and cut into 1 inch pieces
- 12 tbsp mustard oil

- 6 tbsp ginger coarsely ground
- 4 tbsp garlic coarsely ground
- 1½ tbsp mustard seeds powdered
- 1½ tbsp Kashmiri red chilli powder
- 1½ tbsp garam masala powder
- 1 cup jaggery (grated)
- 2 tbsp salt
- 3 tbsp white vinegar with mother

Method:

1. Heat the oil in a non-stick wok.
2. Add the coarsely ground ginger and garlic and sauté till light golden.
3. Add the powdered mustard seeds, red chilli powder and garam masala powder, and sauté for a few seconds. Add the jaggery and salt and mix well.
4. Add the vegetables, mix well and cook for 3–4 minutes.
5. Take the pan off the heat and set aside to cool completely.
6. Stir in the vinegar and mix well.
7. Store in sterilized bottles. This pickle will keep for one year.

Notes:

- As unripe and raw vegetables are used for the making of pickles, their antioxidant content is kept intact.
- Pickles prepared using salt and natural methods can lead to the growth of probiotics or friendly bacteria in digestion.
- Freshly-made pickles are rich in vitamin A, C, K, folates and essential minerals like calcium, iron

and potassium that protect the body from several diseases.

- Pickles are high on salt which increases the risk of hypertension and also heart disease. The main risk of eating pickles is an increase in blood pressure.

Luke's Immunity-Boosting Powder

A simple home-made powder made from specific spices that have immunity-boosting properties.

- A delicious and versatile immunity booster.
- Perfect for cold and flu season.
- Safe for kids.

You can make this powerful immunity-boosting powder with spices that are already lying in your kitchen cabinet. Make them for your house help, drivers, building watchmen, security guards too, or simply share this recipe with them.

Ingredients:

- 7 tbsp organic turmeric powder
- 4 tbsp cumin seeds
- 4 tbsp coriander seeds
- 7 tbsp fennel seeds
- 2 tbsp dry ginger powder
- 2 tbsp whole black pepper
- ½ tbsp Sri Lankan rolled cinnamon powder
- 3 tbsp cardamom powder/pods

Method:

1. Keep turmeric powder and dry ginger powder in a separate bowl (no roasting).

2. Lightly roast all the remaining ingredients on a low flame till you get a nice aroma (avoid burning).

3. Once cooled, transfer them to a grinder and grind to a powder.

4. Add turmeric and dry ginger powder to it and mix with a dry spoon.

5. Store in a clean, airtight glass or steel jar.

How to consume

- Have ¼–1 tsp with a glass of warm water in the morning or mix ¼–1 tsp of the mix in some organic A2 ghee and have it off the spoon. A good fat source always helps enhance adsorption. Generally, 5 gm a day is safe.

- You can add it to your bowl of piping hot soup while cooking it or to your kadhi, rasam, sambar or any curry or sabji. You can also use it to make your pulaos and khichdis. Use it the way you would use your spices while cooking.

- It makes for a great alternative to garam masala as well.

- Use it as seasoning.

Who can consume it?

Anyone and everyone can consume it to boost immunity—the biggest investment today. It's great for your kids and the elderly. Mothers of young kids can mix it in small quantities in their food—like dals, soups, khichdi and porridge. You can consume it every day or when you feel your health is dipping. If you cannot make the mix at home, then you can always get your hands on the readymade immunity boosting powder, for your convenience.

Chutney Corner

Power packed	Flax seeds	Moringa	Curry leaves	Garlic
• ½ cup pumpkin seeds (soaked for 5–6 hours) • ½ cup fresh coriander/ mint leaves	• ½ cup raw flax seeds • 2 dry red chillies • ½ cup fresh grated coconut • 2 tbsp sesame seeds	• ½ cup washed moringa leaves • ¼ cup fresh grated coconut • 1 tbsp tamarind	• 1 cup curry leaves • 1 tbsp urad dal	• 1 large bulb of garlic cloves, peeled and chopped • 1 large tomato, diced

Method:

To any chutney add 1 tsp cumin seeds, a pinch of pink salt and 2 tbsp water.

Snacks

Even though snacking is considered unhealthy, snacks can be an important part of your diet. They can provide energy in the middle of the day or when you exercise. A healthy snack between meals also decreases hunger and keeps you from overeating at mealtime.

1. Kachri
2. Fermented Rice Porridge

Kachri

Water chestnuts usually make an appearance with the onset of winter. This hot and spicy snack is also perfect during the monsoon. Kachri is a famous street-side delicacy from the by-lanes of Uttar Pradesh and Uttarakhand. During winters, a steaming bowl of homemade kachri can be expected any time from the next door neighbour's kitchen as a kind and warm gesture.

The water chestnuts used for this recipe are the dark purple ones and not the green ones. They are boiled and then cooked over low flame till they are ready to be served. The kachri is then served with vibrant and bold chutneys, chopped onion and cilantro to complete the flavourful experience.

Ingredients:

1. 75 gm water chestnuts
2. Salt to taste
3. 1 tsp oil
4. 1 tsp asafoetida
5. 2 tsp cumin powder
6. ½ tsp red chilli powder
7. 1 green chilli finely chopped
8. 1 inch ginger peeled and grated
9. Juice of 1 lemon

Method:

1. Wash the water chestnuts.
2. Pressure cook them with salt for one or two whistles over medium heat. Turn off the heat. Let the steam release naturally from the pressure cooker.
3. Now it becomes easy to remove the outer peel of water chestnut. Collect the pale white pulp in a separate bowl.
4. Add salt, chilli powder, cumin powder over the boiled water chestnuts. Mash completely using a potato

masher. The mashed water chestnuts will be similar to the stuffing for aloo paratha.

5. Heat butter in a heavy bottom pan over medium heat.

6. Now add asafoetida, grated ginger and green chilli. Sauté for a few seconds or till the aroma of ginger is released.

7. Add mashed water chestnuts and roast over low heat till the mixture turns pale brown in colour and starts leaving the sides of the pan. Keep stirring the mixture while it is roasting. Slow cooking is the trick behind making the perfect kachri.

8. Once the kachri is nicely roasted, a pleasant aroma is released. The taste and texture of the mixture is also refined. Taste and adjust seasoning accordingly.

9. Before serving, drizzle lemon juice, sprinkle chopped coriander and pour a teaspoon of melted butter on top.

10. Serve singhare ki kachri warm with coriander chutney.

Nutrition Table:

Calories (kcal)	Carbohydrates (g)	Protein (g)	Fat (g)
107	16	0.6	5

Fermented Rice Porridge

Ingredients:

1. 1 cup cooked whole rice

2. 2 cups water

3. Tempering of your choice (onions, green chillies, ginger chilli paste, mustard and curry leaves)

4. A pinch of salt

Method:

Soak the cooked rice overnight in water. The next day, mix the water and rice. Add seasoning to make a surprisingly filling porridge and enjoy.

Serves 1–2

Benefits:

- It is known to prevent constipation, and because of the high fibre content of the grains, it also clears bowel movement. The starch from the rice or grain water will stimulate the growth of useful bacteria that help with digestion.

- In Indian homes, rice kanji is often used as a remedy for fever. It prevents water loss caused due to vomiting and speeds up the recovery process.

- Rice water is also a great home remedy for treating diarrhoea. Since infants are prone to this digestive problem, they are often given rice water to replenish lost water content. In fact, a study has found that rice water is more effective in controlling diarrhoea by reducing the volume and frequency of stool output in babies.

Nutrition Table:

Calories (kcal)	Carbohydrates (g)	Protein (g)	Fat (g)
100	22	2.1	0.2

Sweets

Sweet snacks increase our production of the so-called hormone of happiness.

1. Tilpita
2. Ande ka Halwa

3. Gondh Laddoo
4. Panjiri
5. Makhana Kheer

Tilpita

Sesame pancakes cooked during the Bihu festival in Assam.

Ingredients:

- 1 cup sticky rice
- 2 cups jaggery
- 1 cup sesame seeds
- 1 tbsp dried coconut
- 2 tbsp fennel seeds

Method:

1. Grind the soaked sticky rice.
2. Cover it and freeze overnight to prepare a flour.
3. To prepare stuffing: Add dried coconut and fennel seeds in jaggery and mix them using your hands.
4. Spread rice powder on a tawa and keep it for 2–3 seconds. Add stuffing in the middle. Use a fork to roll.
5. It is ready and can be stored for 2–3 weeks.

Notes:

- The recipe is a great source of nutrients and is a treat for those with a sweet tooth.
- Sesame seeds are high in magnesium, which helps lower blood pressure.
- Lignans, vitamin E and other antioxidants in sesame seeds help prevent plaque build-up in your arteries.

- Sesame seeds, both un-hulled and hulled, are rich in several nutrients that boost bone health.

- Sesame seeds are a good source of thiamine, niacin and vitamin B6, which are necessary for proper cellular function and metabolism.

- Sesame seeds also supply iron, copper and vitamin B6, needed for blood cell formation and function.

- The lignans in sesame seeds function as antioxidants, which help fight oxidative stress—a chemical reaction that may damage your cells and increase the risk of many chronic diseases.

- Sesame seeds are a good source of several nutrients including zinc, selenium, copper, iron, vitamin B6 and vitamin E that are important for immune system function.

- Sesamin, a compound in sesame seeds, may help reduce joint pain and support mobility in arthritis of the knee.

- Sesame seeds are good sources of nutrients such as selenium, iron, copper, zinc and vitamin B6 that support thyroid health.

Nutrition Table:

Calories (kcal)	Carbohydrates (g)	Protein (g)	Fat (g)
150	15	4	8.2

Ande ka Halwa

Halwa is one of the most popular desserts in India. There are a number of variants depending on the ingredients used; gajar ka halwa, suji ka halwa or lauki ka halwa. You may have heard of or eaten all of them if you belong to a typical Indian family. Usually, these delicacies are prepared during the festive season. While halwa is a very common dessert for Indians, there is a variant that most people haven't had the pleasure of tasting yet.

Ingredients:

- 100 ml A2 milk/almond milk
- 2 eggs
- 2 tbsp powdered organic jaggery
- A pinch of crushed cardamom
- 1 tbsp ghee
- Almonds, cashews, and raisins

Method:

1. Break the eggs and keep in a bowl.
2. Add milk and powdered organic jaggery and stir.
3. Heat ghee in a pan on low flame and pour in the egg mixture.
4. Cook on low flame till it starts to solidify.
5. A very sweet aroma of ghee and eggs will spread; add chopped cashews, almonds and raisins.
6. Switch off the gas before it gets too thick.
7. Serve hot (serves 4–5).

Notes:

- This recipe is excellent for fitness enthusiasts.
- Eggs are considered one of the most perfect sources of protein.
- Eggs are the perfect source of dietary vitamin D. Vitamin D is essential for bone health, but it is also a vitamin that we cannot synthesize on our own, so we are dependent on outside sources to keep us strong.
- Eggs are one of the richest dietary sources of choline.

Choline is a macronutrient that is essential for several important physiological functions including neurological development, nerve function, muscle control and metabolism.

- Rich source of lutein and zeaxanthin, key nutrients for good eye health.

Nutrition Table:

Calories (kcal)	Carbohydrates (g)	Protein (g)	Fat (g)
127	16	5.7	4.5

Gondh Laddoo

Ingredients:

- 150 gm gondh (edible gum)
- 350 gm ghee
- 400 gm whole wheat flour/jowar/bajra
- 400 gm powdered jaggery
- 50 gm dry coconut
- 50 gm chopped almonds
- 50 gm chopped cashew nuts (optional)

Method:

1. In a large and heavy-bottomed pan, add 350 gm ghee and melt on a low flame.
2. Once the ghee melts, add gondh to the pan, a little at a time, and shallow fry on low flame until the gondh puffs up like popcorn and turns crispy.
3. Make sure that the gondh is completely cooked from the inside and outside. Repeat the process with rest of the gondh.

4. Once the gondh is fried, using a ladle, separate the gondh from the ghee and keep aside to cool down.

5. In the same pan containing the melted ghee, add whole wheat flour and roast until it becomes aromatic and brown. The mixture should be crumbly. Turn off the flame.

6. Transfer the flour on to a plate. Add the powdered jaggery and all the dry fruits and mix well. Let the mixture cool down.

7. Once the gondh has cooled, with a rolling pin, crush it into a coarse powder. Add this crushed gondh to the dry fruits and flour mixture.

8. Now take a little amount of the mixture in your hands and give it a round shape.

9. Keep the laddoos aside for a few hours; they will set properly. You can keep them in an airtight container for a month.

Notes:

- A single gondh laddoo will provide energy that will last for hours.

- Gondh laddoos are given to lactating mothers too as it is said to increase the production of breast milk.

- It has purgative properties and hence, is effective for treating constipation.

- Gondh is helpful in regaining strength and helps a mother to cope with the challenges of motherhood.

- It also helps to control heavy blood flow during periods.

- It increases libido and is also useful for treating sexual inadequacy or weakness in men.

- It has anti-ageing properties that are beneficial for your skin as it delays the development of wrinkles and fine lines.

- It is a part of herbal treatment for women who have small breasts and wish to increase their size.
- It helps delay wrinkles and fine lines.

Nutrition Table:

Calories (kcal)	Carbohydrates (g)	Protein (g)	Fat (g)
248	35	4.5	10

Panjiri (Gluten-free)

Ingredients:

- 1 cup sattu flour
- 1 cup finger millet flour or steel-cut oats
- ½ cup ethically sourced A2 ghee
- Mixed nuts—almonds and unsalted pistachios (those with a nut allergy can skip this ingredient)
- 1 tbsp sesame seeds, roasted and powdered
- 1 tbsp pumpkin seeds
- 2 tbsp edible gum (gondh), fried and coarsely powdered
- 1 tbsp ground flaxseed powder
- ¼ cup fox nuts, roasted and powdered
- 1 tsp ginger powder
- 1 tsp cardamom powder
- 1 cup organic jaggery
- ¼ tsp fenugreek seed powder

Method:

1. Grind roasted oats into a powder.
2. Separately grind the nuts and seeds (pre-soaked, dried and powdered) and keep aside.
3. Take 1 tbsp A2 ghee in a pan, roast the makhanas, powder once it cools down, and keep them aside.
4. In a pan, add the remaining ghee, powdered oats and sattu flour. Stir it well till a mild aroma is released and the mixture turns semi-brown in colour.
5. Add nuts and seeds, ginger powder, gondh, cardamom powder, crushed makhanas, sesame seeds powder, ground flax and methi powder.
6. Stir in all the ingredients well on slow gas for 3 minutes.
7. Turn off the gas.
8. Add jaggery powder and mix well.
9. Allow the mixture to cool down.
10. Store in airtight containers.

Variations:

1. One can add amaranth flour or roasted poha powder in place of the ragi flour.
2. Sattu flour can be replaced by moong flour.
3. For sweetness, one can consider date palm jaggery.
4. Adding grated coconut will further enhance the taste and flavour.
5. Use it in porridge form, or add it to milk, or roll it into small laddoos.
6. One can also make pancakes by adding almond milk!

Notes:

- Panjiri is a winter immunity-booster.
- It is anti-inflammatory and is often eaten in winters to replenish and strengthen the body.
- Having panjiri after a delivery is extremely helpful for a new mother, as it has healing properties and also stimulates lactation.
- The ingredients used to make panjiri have adaptogenic properties that help the body repair and heal itself.
- Panjiri is rich in calcium, iron, protein, healthy fats and fibre.

Nutrition Table:

Calories (kcal)	Carbohydrates (g)	Protein (g)	Fat (g)
160	15	6.5	12

Makhana Kheer

Ingredients:

- 1½ cup unsweetened almond milk
- 1 cup roasted makhana (fox nuts)
- 1 tsp pure saffron
- 3 tbsp chopped nuts (almonds, pistachios)
- 2 tsp pumpkin seeds (to garnish)
- 1 tbsp jaggery powder or 2 tbsp date puree made at home

Method:

1. Heat the almond milk.
2. Once it starts boiling, add saffron and nuts.

3. Now add the makhana.
4. Give it 2 boils.
5. Add the nuts and jaggery/date puree.
6. Turn off the gas.
7. Garnish with pumpkin seeds.
8. Serve hot.

Notes:

- Makhana is rich in calcium, protein and magnesium.
- Almond milk is rich in vitamin E, magnesium, calcium, good fats and protein.

Nutrition Table:

Calories (kcal)	Carbohydrates (g)	Protein (g)	Fat (g)
169	20	7.5	6.5

Staples

Food staples are eaten regularly—even daily—and supply a major proportion of a person's energy and nutritional needs. Food staples vary from place to place, depending on the food sources available.

1. Makhana Paratha
2. Doli ki Roti
3. Sattu Methi Bhakri

Makhana Paratha

Ingredients:

- 1 cup amaranth/jowar/sattu flour as per choice

- 1 cup (heaped) phool makhana/fox nuts
- 1 generous pinch turmeric powder
- 1 tsp black pepper powder
- ¼ tsp roasted jeera powder
- 2 tbsp coriander/methi/spinach leaves (finely chopped), as per availability
- Rock salt, to taste
- ½ tsp ghee
- Cold pressed coconut oil, to toast parathas

Method:

1. Heat ghee in a skillet, add makhana and roast till golden or until crispy. Once it's crispy and not chewy, that's the right stage. Switch off and cool down.

2. Transfer it to a mixer jar and grind it to a fine powder.

3. In another mixing bowl, take all other ingredients (except oil) along with makhana powder.

4. First mix well with a spoon, then add water and knead it to a soft pliable dough. Allow it to rest for 15 minutes at least.

5. Then knead again and form lemon-sized balls.

6. Take a ball and start rolling. Dust flour if needed, to avoid sticking.

7. Roll thin parathas. Roll the rest of the parathas too and keep them ready.

8. Heat a dosa tawa, drizzle oil and then carefully transfer the paratha.

9. Cook till small bubbles starts to appear, then flip to the other side. Drizzle a little oil/ghee and cook until brown spots appear here and there. Flip again if needed.

10. Serve hot.

Notes:

- Makhana/lotus seeds are an extremely good source of manganese, potassium, magnesium, thiamine, protein and phosphorus.
- Amaranth flour is versatile, full of whole-grain nutrition and is used during fasting, too.
- It contains all the nine essential amino acids and lysine, a protein missing in most grains.
- Amaranth is a good source of iron, magnesium, calcium and phosphorus.

Nutrition Table:

Calories (kcal)	Carbohydrates (g)	Protein (g)	Fat (g)
145	19.3	5.7	5

Doli ki Roti

Doli ki roti is an indigenously fermented bread commonly prepared by the Indian Punjabi community. Doli is an earthen pot and roti means bread, hence the name. This fermented product is based on the natural fermentation of wheat flour along with spice mixture. The final product is a puri stuffed with legumes. This contains good amounts of protein, fat, fibre and minerals, and reduces anti-nutrients. A whole wheat fermented roti, activated with an age-old, traditional recipe of homemade yeast.

Ingredients:

For water to create yeast:
- 5 black cardamoms
- ¼ cup fennel seeds

- ¼ cup Bengal gram dal
- ¼ cup khus khus, or poppy seeds
- ¼ cup mishri
- 250 ml water (1 cup)

For homemade yeast:

- 2 tsp whole wheat flour

For roti:

- 2 cups whole wheat flour
- 1 tsp jaggery
- ½ tsp salt

Lukewarm water (to knead)

- Cooking oil, to deep fry

For filling:

- 1 cup Bengal gram dal
- Salt to taste
- ½ tsp red chilli powder (adjust accordingly)
- 1 tsp coriander powder
- ½ tsp Luke's Immunity-Boosting Powder
- 1 tsp organic turmeric powder
- 1 inch crushed ginger
- ¼ cup onion (finely chopped)
- Water, as needed

Method:

1. In a saucepan, add water (250 ml) and bring to a boil. Add all the ingredients listed in the 'For water to create yeast' list above.

2. Cover and boil for 2 minutes until mishri dissolves

and the chana dal softens a bit. Let it remain covered. Wrap this saucepan in a dry and warm cloth and keep in the warmest corner of your kitchen undisturbed for 24 hours.

3. To prepare yeast, take the frothy water after 24 hours (only if it is frothy, or you need to keep it for a few more hours/repeat the procedure) to prepare homemade yeast. Pass the water through a sieve and mix it with whole wheat flour (3 tbsp). The batter should resemble pancake batter. Cover it again with a lid, wrap with a warm cloth and keep in a warm place for 3 more hours.

4. After 3 hours, the mixture will seem bubbly and frothy. Now you may proceed with making the dough. Take the homemade yeast mixture and add the ingredients from the roti ingredient list and knead to make a smooth pliable dough. Use only warm water to knead the dough. Keep it covered like before, for 3 hours or just 30 minutes more, until it rises.

For the filling:

1. Clean chana dal and pressure cook adding salt, turmeric, ginger with a little water for 2 whistles or till cooked soft; drain the remaining water completely and discard.

2. Once the dal is cooled a bit, add spices and onion, mix well.

For Doli ki Roti:

1. Heat oil in a deep frying pan on medium heat.
2. Roll out a roti stuffed with chana dal (like a paratha).
3. Shallow fry.
4. Drain on a kitchen towel.

5. Repeat till all the dough and filling is used.
6. Serve doli ki roti with a bowl of A2 milk curd.

Notes:

- The antinutrients like phytic acid and trypsin inhibitors are present in considerable amounts in the unfermented bread, but are reduced to the extent of 5 to 18 per cent (phytic acid) and 49 to 70 per cent (trypsin inhibitors) due to the fermentation.

- Phytic acid is the major storage form of phosphorus in cereals and pulses. Research indicates that, on fermentation, phytic acid was reduced in Doli ki Roti tremendously.

- Fermentation of the cereal–pulse blend reduces the anti-nutritional factors, phytic acid and increases bio-availability of minerals, iron and calcium.

- Due to a proper blend of cereals and pulses, the biological value of protein content is improved.

- It's a fermented product; hence, excellent for the gut.

- The spices used for fermentation impart a natural flavour and have antimicrobial properties that arrest the growth of pathogenic microflora.

Nutrition Table:

Calories (kcal)	Carbohydrates (g)	Protein (g)	Fat (g)
232	34.5	6.2	8.3

Sattu Methi Bhakri

Sattu is a product of desi chana (black gram), widely used in ancient India and modern India. Sattu is the world's oldest instant food. From the Himalayas to the plains of Asia, sattu can be readily consumed without any fuel, utensils, vegetables or cooking oils. No other product can beat it. Just mix sattu with water to prepare an instant nourishing drink. Since sattu is protein-rich and oil-free, physicians recommend it to all types of diabetes patients. Sattu helps to build muscle mass and keeps the body fit and healthy.

Sattu Methi Bhakri is one of the easiest and most nutritious dishes one can have for breakfast or as a snack. It is actually a roti rolled out by combining sattu flour with fenugreek leaves and other ingredients.

Ingredients:

- 1 cup sattu flour
- ½ cup fenugreek leaves (finely chopped)
- 1 green chilli (chopped)
- ½ tsp ajwain
- ¼ tsp turmeric powder
- Lukewarm water to bind (as per requirement)
- Oil, as required (can use cold pressed coconut oil)
- Salt, as per taste (pink Himalayan salt)

Method:

1. To prepare methi bhakri, mix sattu, fenugreek leaves, green chilli, ajwain, salt, 1 tbsp oil and turmeric powder.
2. Knead it well along with a little lukewarm water to make a hard dough.
3. Roll them out a little thicker than the usual rotis.
4. Place them on a griddle and cook both sides by applying a little oil or ghee.

Notes:

- Methi bhakri is unique and tasty with an appetizing

methi flavour and aroma. Methi adds to the fibre content and is useful for managing blood sugar levels.

- Sattu is a great Indian protein source, high on soluble fibre, low on glycaemic index and easier to digest. It's rich in minerals like iron, manganese, molybdenum, zinc, magnesium and calcium.

- Methi bhakri should be carefully rolled out. It should be thick so that it doesn't fall apart. Make sure the dough is not watery at all.

- Adding ajwain makes it highly beneficial for the digestive system because of its carminative properties.

Nutrition Table:

Calories (kcal)	Carbohydrates (g)	Protein (g)	Fat (g)
154	19	8.2	5

Gravies/Dal/Vegetables

Indians should be proud of their curry. Any Indian food that is cooked and served the right way, and within the framework of the laws of nature, is one of the best healing cuisines. It isn't fair to say it is the best in the world, because each country must embrace its traditional food and culture. However, this is best suited for Indians.

The beauty of Indian curry is the synergy between two or more ingredients. There is a lot of wisdom in these combinations. It is nutrient-dense, immunity-boosting, anti-inflammatory, a digestion booster, and by itself, a natural medicine for many ailments. It is when we replace traditional wisdom with junk, processed, and so-called fast and convenient foods, that we become deficient in nutrients, and these deficiencies lead to all the ailments.

1. Besan Kadhi

2. Sarson ka Saag
3. Harive Soppu Bendi
4. Tere Tonak: Goan Colocasia Leaf Curry
5. Dai-Nei-Iong
6. Tripuri Muya Awandru

Besan Kadhi

Ingredients:

- 3 cups A2 yoghurt
- 1 cup roasted sattu flour
- 1 tsp turmeric powder
- 1 tsp chilli powder
- Salt to taste
- 1 tsp garam masala/immunity powder
- 10–12 peanuts (semi-boiled)
- 6 cups water
- 2 tsp coconut oil/A2 ghee
- ½ tsp asafoetida
- 2 tsp cumin seeds
- 2 whole red chillies
- ½ tsp mustard seeds
- 2 tsp urad dal

Method:

1. Mix the roasted sattu flour, turmeric, chilli powder, salt and garam masala.
2. Add yoghurt gradually to this mixture to form a smooth paste, and then add water.

3. Heat the oil in a large pan; add the asafoetida, cumin seeds, mustard seeds, urad dal and whole red chillies.

4. When the mustard seeds begin to splutter, add the flour and yoghurt mixture, peanuts and bring to a boil.

5. Add salt as per taste.

6. Simmer over a low heat till it thickens.

7. Garnish with coriander.

8. Serve hot (serves 4).

Notes:

- Loaded with vitamins and minerals, Besan Kadhi is perfect for improving body functions and growth. It is primarily rich in protein, calcium and phosphorus.

- Goodbye anaemia. No more fatigue; iron and protein are the perfect combination to increase haemoglobin.

- Hello to healthy skin and hair. Be it acne, dark spots or any skin issue, besan boosts collagen formation and has anti-inflammatory properties.

- Can be consumed during pregnancy. Folate? Present! Vitamin B6? Present! Iron? Present! Baby growth, yes! Chances of miscarriage, reduced!

- Loaded with good bacteria for the gut. Maintains gut-flora and helps in nutrient absorption.

- Besan and curd, both rich in calcium, make it friendly for healthy bones. Additionally, phosphorus makes it perfect as phosphorus combines with calcium to build bones and teeth.

- Rich in magnesium, causes the muscles to relax and hence, maintains heart health. While phosphorus regulates lipid mechanism.

- Since it is low in the glycaemic index, it's perfect for

people with diabetes. Reduces blood sugar and insulin.

Nutrition Table:

Calories (kcal)	Carbohydrates (g)	Protein (g)	Fat (g)
159	28	8.9	8.6

Variation: Vegan Kadhi using coconut milk and sattu as main ingredients.

Sarson ka Saag

This famous recipe from north India is made with a combination of greens and a dash of spices that add more zing to this delicious sabji, making it a treat for the taste buds. Serve this delicious Sarson ka Saag with Makai ki Roti, to make a satiating north Indian meal.

Ingredients:

- 2½ cups washed and chopped mustard leaves
- 1 cup washed and chopped spinach
- 1 cup bathua leaves
- 1 cup radish leaves
- 1–2 roughly chopped green chillies
- ½ tbsp oil
- ½ tsp cumin seeds
- ½ tbsp finely chopped garlic
- ½ tbsp finely chopped ginger
- ¼ cup finely chopped onions
- ½ cup tomatoes (optional)
- ⅛ tsp asafoetida
- ¼ tsp turmeric powder
- ½ tsp chilli powder

- ½ tsp coriander-cumin seeds powder (optional)
- Salt to taste

Method:

1. Boil enough water in a deep non-stick pan, add the mustard leaves, spinach, bathua and radish leaves and green chillies, mix well and cook on a high flame for 4–5 minutes, while stirring occasionally.

2. Strain using a strainer and drain well.

3. Refresh it twice in cold water immediately and drain well again. Keep aside for 2–3 minutes to cool slightly.

4. Blend in a mixer to a coarse mixture using ½ cup of water. Keep aside.

5. Heat the oil in a non-stick kadai and add the cumin seeds.

6. When the seeds crackle, add the garlic, ginger and asafoetida and sauté on a medium flame for 30 seconds.

7. Add the onions and sauté again on a medium flame for 1 to 2 minutes.

8. Add the mustard leaves-spinach mixture, turmeric powder, chilli powder, coriander-cumin seeds powder and salt, mix well and cook on a medium flame for 2–3 minutes, while stirring occasionally.

9. Serve hot with Makai ki Roti.

Notes:

- The main ingredient, mustard leaves, are rich in anti-cancer nutrients and also help lower blood cholesterol levels.

- Spinach is a good source of fibre and is loaded with magnesium, which is needed for healthy nerves and muscles.

- Bathua leaves are rich in fibre and water content, cure constipation (due to their laxative properties) and a host of your tummy problems by aiding digestion and boosting intestinal activity, too.

- Bathua's role in keeping your liver healthy has made these lovely greens a hit in the health and nutrition circuit.

- Radish leaves are an excellent detoxifying agent and also help in the digestive process.

- Ginger, garlic and onions, which are used in this dish, have anti-inflammatory benefits and are very high in antioxidants.

- Mustard leaves may increase brain dopamine levels. Also improve cognitive and other functions of the central nervous system.

Nutrition Table:

Calories (kcal)	Carbs (g)	Protein (g)	Fat (g)	Calcium	Iron	Fibre (g)
80	7.8	5.4	5.9	344	356	4.8

Harive Soppu Bendi

Harive Soppu Bendi is the traditional name of this dish. Bendi is a simple, mildly spiced coconut gravy made using gourds like bottle gourd, pumpkin, ash gourd or greens like spinach, malabar spinach, green/red amaranth, etc. The only spice used in the coconut gravy is cumin and a green chilli or two for a light kick of heat. Harive Soppu Bendi makes a perfect curry for little ones or those who can't handle very spicy curries. With no overpowering spices competing, the naturally astringent flavour of amaranth leaves comes through the mild coconut gravy. Try this simple and flavourful amaranth coconut curry when you feel like eating some light and healthy food and your taste buds will thank you!

Ingredients:

- 1 bunch tender harive soppu/green amaranth leaves (around 2½–3 packed cups)
- 1 tsp jaggery
- Salt to taste

For coconut paste:

- 1½ packed cups grated coconut (fresh or frozen)
- 1 tsp cumin seeds
- 1–2 green chillies (slit)

For tadka/tempering:

- 1 tsp mustard seeds
- 1 dry red chilli, cut into 2–3 pieces
- A pinch of asafoetida (optional)
- A sprig of curry leaves
- ½ tbsp oil (preferably coconut oil)

Method:

1. Clean and wash the tender amaranth leaves by soaking them in a bowl of water with a tsp of salt for 10–15 minutes. This helps in cleaning any residues of pesticides clinging to the leaves. After they have been thoroughly washed, chop them into strips of 1 inch thickness. Use the tender stems as well, and cut them into 1 inch long pieces. Set aside until needed.

2. Cook the amaranth leaves in 1 cup of water along with the stems, jaggery and salt to taste. Cook it only until they wilt and don't lose their vibrant green colour; thus

about 3 minutes.

3. While the leaves are getting cooked, grind grated coconut along with cumin seeds and green chillies by adding a little water to make a smooth and thick paste.

4. Add this coconut paste to the cooked greens and reduce the heat to low. Adjust the salt and let it cook uncovered until small bubbles start to appear on surface, about 5–7 minutes, and turn off the heat.

5. While the curry is simmering, prepare the tadka by heating oil in small pan. Once the oil is hot, add mustard seeds, red chilli pieces and hing. When the mustard seeds start to pop and splutter, add curry leaves and turn off the gas.

6. Transfer the tadka to the Harive Soppu Bendi and mix them well. Cover and let it sit for 10–15 minutes for the flavours to develop and blend well.

7. Serve this delicious and healthy Harive Soppu Bendi with a bowl of steaming rice.

Notes:

- If you are not using home-grown greens or those from organic shops and instead have bought it from the market, it is best to soak it in a bowl of water with a tsp of salt for 10–15 minutes. This helps in cleaning any pesticide residue clinging to the leaves.

- Do not cook this curry for long as it will lose its flavours.

- If you don't get amaranth leaves in your neck of the woods, just replace it with spinach and follow the recipe.

- Amaranth leaves are available in a range of colours from red to green, pink to gold. They are common green leafy vegetables and they grow throughout the country, from the Himalayas to the coastal regions of south India.

- With their higher protein, iron and calcium content, the seeds and leaves have been used by Indians in traditional medicine and cooking for years!
- These leaves help build a good immune system.
- The amaranth leaves are a natural home remedy for hair loss and premature greying as well as for treating skin problems like eczema.
- Along with amaranth leaves, the seeds are effective in treating diarrhoea and excessive menstruation. No wonder that amaranth seeds have been declared as the next 'wondergrain' in the Western world.

Nutrition Table:

Calories (kcal)	Carbohydrates (g)	Protein (g)	Fat (g)
116	1.1	1.9	12

Tere Tonak (Goan Colocasia Leaf Curry)

Ingredients:

- 15–20 colocasia leaves
- ¼ cup chana dal
- 4 peeled and crushed jackfruit seeds

For the masala curry:

- ½ cup freshly grated coconut
- 1 tsp coriander seeds
- ½ tsp turmeric powder
- 3 dry red chillies/shepda/byadgi chillies
- 1 marble-sized ball of tamarind

- 1 tbsp grated jaggery
- 3 kokum petals
- Salt to taste

For tempering:

- 1 tsp mustard seeds
- 1 sprig curry leaves

Method:

1. Before making the colocasia leaves curry, apply oil to your hands and start peeling the stems. Finely chop the stems and leaves.

2. Wash and soak the gram or chana dal for at least 30 minutes.

3. After 30 minutes, take a pressure cooker and add the chopped leaves, stems, chopped jackfruit seeds and gram dal. Add ½ cup water.

4. Pressure cook for 5 whistles or till the gram dal is cooked. Switch off the gas and wait for the natural release of pressure from the cooker.

5. Take a grinder and add all the ingredients meant for the masala gravy, except salt.

6. Add ½ cup water and grind into a thin gravy.

7. Now heat a kadai/heavy-bottomed pan. Add 1 tsp oil. After the oil is heated, add mustard seeds. After mustard seeds splutter, add curry leaves and fry for 30 seconds. Pour the gravy in.

8. Mix the contents from the cooker in the gravy well.

9. Add jaggery and mix. Add kokum petals.

10. Let it simmer.

11. Now add salt to taste and mix.

12. Serve hot with rotis or rice.

Notes:

- Since these colocasia leaves are acrid, some people might get allergic and one's mouth, lips and throat might start itching. So it is always advisable to cook these leaves with a souring agent like tamarind or kokum. Also if you are sensitive, apply oil on your hands before peeling or cutting the leaves.

- Colocasia leaves are rich in vitamin C which acts as an antioxidant. This will help prevent many diseases.

- Vitamin C in 1 cup of taro leaves (145 mg) can reach 86 per cent of the daily value the body needs and vitamin C has a role in improving immunity.

- Colocasia leaves are rich in vitamin A. 1 cup comprises a daily value of 123 per cent which is very good for keeping your eyes healthy.

- Colocasia leaves are high in dietary fibre that helps to absorb and digest food well. Taro leaves can make you stay away from digestive problems such as indigestion, constipation, and also diarrhoea.

- Good fibre content can reduce cholesterol effectively by binding and breaking down fat and cholesterol.

- Colocasia leaves contain vitamin B complex including thiamin, riboflavin, niacin and vitamin B6 that protect the nervous system.

- It is rich in folate which is essential especially during pregnancy for the development of the foetal brain and nervous system. Besides its folate content which is beneficial for the foetus, taro leaves also contain manganese. This mineral helps in the formation of foetal cartilage, bone and teeth during pregnancy.

- Colocasia leaves contain iron which helps in red blood

cell formation. In addition, its vitamin C content helps absorb the iron well. This will meet the need of red blood cells in the body and thus anaemia can be prevented.

Nutrition Table:

Calories (kcal)	Carbohydrates (g)	Protein (g)	Fat (g)
114	12	4	7

Dai-Nei-Iong

Pronounced Dai-Nei-Iong, this is a Khasi dish from the north-east state of Meghalaya. It is a lentil preparation with black sesame seeds.

Ingredients:

- ½ cup brown masoor dal
- ½ cup toor dal
- 2 cups water
- 1 tsp salt
- 1 tsp ginger garlic paste
- 1 tbsp black sesame seeds
- 1 tsp oil
- 1 tsp paprika

Method:

1. Heat a pan and dry roast the sesame seeds for two minutes.
2. Once they start to splutter, turn off the flame and allow it to cool.
3. Grind into a coarse powder without adding any water.

4. Meanwhile, add the dal in a pressure cooker with 2 cups of water for 3 whistles, and release the pressure.

5. Once the pressure is released, mash the dal completely.

6. Heat the kadai and add oil. Once the oil is hot, add the ginger garlic paste.

7. Sauté for a minute and add the cooked dal, powdered sesame seeds, paprika and salt.

8. Mix them all and let it simmer for 5 minutes.

9. Serve hot.

Notes:

- Black gram, being rich in iron and protein, acts as an excellent energy booster.

- Black gram contains magnesium, fibre, folate and potassium that helps keep your heart healthy.

- Dietary fibre is an effective way to control your cholesterol levels, while magnesium helps with blood circulation, and potassium acts as a vasodilator by lowering the tension in blood vessels and arteries.

- In addition, folate is linked with lowering the risk of heart disease.

- Since ancient times, black gram has been used in Ayurvedic medicines for relieving pain and inflammation.

- The presence of antioxidants in black gram is known to reduce pain and inflammation in the body.

- Good source of calcium.

- Improves cognitive function.

Nutrition Table:

Calories (kcal)	Carbohydrates (g)	Protein (g)	Fat (g)
158	18	8	6

Tripuri Muya Awandru

Muya Awandru is boiled bamboo shoot in a rice flour gravy, cooked with fermented fish, green chilli pepper and parsley. Intrinsic to Tripura, this dish is unlike the other spicy dishes of the state, and doesn't require any oil. Bamboo shoots are a nutritive boon for north-east India.

Ingredients:

- 400 gm muya (bamboo) shoots, peel the hard shells until you reach the white and tender shoots and cut into thick round slices or 3 cm long pieces
- 2 tbsp rice flour, coarsely ground
- 2 medium-size fermented fish or 1 cup moong dal
- 1 tsp ginger (chopped) or 3–4 garlic pods (crushed)
- 3–4 green chilli peppers, slit lengthwise
- Salt to taste
- 800 ml water for cooking
- Basil leaves for garnishing

Method:

1. Wash the peeled and cut bamboo shoots and drain excess water.

2. Pressure-cook bamboo shoots on medium-high heat for 2 whistles and set aside, or you could boil it in a pot for about 30 minutes.

3. Add green chilli peppers, fermented fish or 1 cup

boiled moong, chopped ginger, salt and cook for about 4 minutes. Stir occasionally.

4. Add 2 tbsp of water to the rice flour in a bowl and make a paste. Add this paste as you stir the curry continuously to avoid any rice flour lumps. Cover and let the awandru simmer for another 4–5 minutes.

5. Once done, garnish with basil leaves and enjoy it hot with rice.

Notes:

- Fermented fish provides the body with iron and phosphorus, and there is also a decrease in the phytate content in these fermented products.
- Bamboo shoot is low in calories, but has a good amount of protein.
- Bamboo shoot contains vitamin A, vitamin E, B vitamins including vitamin B6, thiamin, riboflavin, niacin, folate and pantothenic acid.
- Bamboo shoot is also rich in calcium, magnesium, phosphorus, potassium, sodium, zinc, copper, manganese, selenium and iron.
- Bamboo shoot possesses anti-inflammatory and analgesic properties. It also works against ulcers.
- Bamboo shoot juice can also be used as a medicine for external wounds and ulcers.
- Bamboo shoot has been known to be effective against respiratory disorders.
- Bamboo leaves are also suggested as a remedy for intestinal worms and stomach disorders.
- Bamboo shoot contains a high amount of potassium. Potassium is highly beneficial as an electrolyte, and is also very good for lowering and maintaining healthy blood pressure.

- It is believed that bamboo extracts contain antivenin properties, in the case of snake or scorpion bites.

Nutrition Table:

Calories (kcal)	Carbohydrates (g)	Protein (g)	Fat (g)
167	24	9	7

One-Pot Meals

Different versions of these dishes span the globe and the defining factor is in the name: it requires only one pot. They contain almost all the nutrients, are easy to prepare, and you don't need any side dishes.

1. Curd Rice
2. Dal Dhokli
3. Gatta Pulao

Curd Rice

Curd rice is a staple dish of south Indian cuisine. It makes a great summer food as well. It is called *Thayir Sadam* in Tamil and *Daddojanam* in Telugu.

Curd contains tryptophan, an amino acid required for the creation of serotonin. Serotonin has a wide variety of functions in the body; it is also a neuro-chemical and a natural mood regulator, that makes us feel happy, emotionally stable, less anxious, more tranquil, and even more focused and energetic. It also plays a role in learning memory and digestion.

Many foods contain tryptophan, but what makes the brain absorb tryptophan to create serotonin is carbohydrates! So it's the combination of tryptophan-containing curd and the carbs in the rice that creates the bliss we experience after eating curd rice! Let's be happy that our ancestors knew these simple ways of creating daily happiness and reach for that pot of curd rice.

Ingredients:

- ½ cup short grain rice
- ½ cup curd
- ¼ cup milk (if you will be consuming it after 7–8 hours)
- 2 tbsp carrot (grated)
- Salt to taste
- 1 tsp oil
- ½ tsp mustard seeds
- 10–12 curry leaves
- 1 tsp urad (black gram) dal
- ½ tsp ginger (grated)
- 1 dry red chilli (broken)
- 1 tbsp fresh coriander (chopped)

Method:

1. Wash the rice and cook with 1½ cup water until fully cooked. Rice should be mushy.
2. Bring the rice to room temperature.
3. Add curd, milk, carrot and salt and mix well.
4. Slightly mash the rice using your hands.
5. Heat oil in a pan.
6. Once the oil is hot, add mustard seeds and curry leaves and let them crackle for a few seconds.
7. Add urad dal, ginger and dry red chillies and fry until dal turns slightly brown.
8. Pour the tempered mixture over curd rice and mix well.

9. Garnish with fresh coriander.
10. Serve chilled.

Notes:

- High biological value protein.
- Curd, being a natural probiotic, is excellent for the gut.
- Curd rice can alleviate upset stomach, diarrhoea, indigestion and bloating.
- Helps cool your body down after a meal loaded with spices.
- If one is on a lot of medication, probiotic supplementation is important to balance microflora.
- When one has fever, curd rice helps cool the body.
- It's good for boosting immunity as it is good for the gut, since 75 per cent of immunity starts in the gut.
- For women undergoing premenstrual syndrome, suffering from pain and bloating, curd rice is a good probiotic. Also, it can help balance your calcium levels. Additionally, the dish is rich in magnesium, vitamin B6 and manganese that can alleviate PMS symptoms. These nutrients may help you feel less depressed, and reduce irritation and moodiness around the time of your period.
- Also, the tempering with mustard seeds, curry leaves, etc. help in expelling excess mucus from the body, thereby keeping your lungs healthy.
- For the ones with stomach ulcers or mouth ulcers, it is an excellent soft and nutritious meal!

Nutrition Table:

Calories (kcal)	Carbohydrates (g)	Protein (g)	Fat (g)
192	27	5.9	8

Dal Dhokli/Indian-style Pasta

A traditional Gujarati dish generally prepared with lentils and wheat flour as base ingredients. It contains soft-textured dhokli submerged in semi-thick lentil gravy and has a mildly sweet and spicy taste of aromatic spices and crunchy peanuts. Apart from being healthy and easy to prepare, this delicious Dal Dhokli is capable of carrying an entire meal on its own!

Ingredients:

For the dal:

- 1 cup toor (pigeon pea) dal
- 2 tbsp peanuts (soaked in water for 30 minutes)
- 5 garlic cloves (chopped)
- 4 kokums
- 1 tsp cumin seeds
- ½ tsp turmeric powder
- ½ tsp chilli powder
- Lemon
- Coriander leaves

For the dhokli:

- 1 cup wheat flour
- ½ tsp asafoetida
- ½ tsp chilli powder
- ½ tsp turmeric

- Oil
- Salt to taste

Method:

1. Boil dal and peanuts in a pressure cooker until soft and keep aside.
2. Heat 1 tbsp ghee in a pan and add cumin seeds, garlic, asafoetida and finally, the boiled dal.
3. Add kokum, turmeric powder, chilli powder, sugar and curry leaves. Boil and add salt to taste.
4. Note: You can add vegetables as well.
5. For dhokli:
6. Mix the flour, salt, turmeric, chilli powder, asafoetida and a little oil and make a stiff dough with water. Knead well and roll out into 10 cm discs.
7. Cut the discs into diamonds or squares with a knife and drop them into the boiling dal mixture.
8. When all the dhokli pieces are in, boil the dal for a further 15 minutes on a low flame. Garnish with coriander leaves and serve hot.

Notes:

- It makes a wholesome/complete vegetarian protein meal.
- The combination of cereal and pulse lowers the GI and GL making it ideal for diabetics.
- Kokum is known as grandma's cure for reducing acidity.
- Kokum is also rich in garcinol imparting antioxidant properties.
- Lemon helps to load vitamin C and hence boosts immunity.
- Coriander leaves are a good source of iron and folate

and, combined with the vitamin C from lemon, help in the absorption of iron from food.

Nutrition Table:

Calories (kcal)	Carbohydrates (g)	Protein (g)	Fat (g)
296	41.6	11	10.3

Gatte ka Pulao

Ingredients:

For besan gatta:

- 1½ cup gram flour
- A pinch of asafoetida
- ¼ tsp turmeric powder
- 1 tsp red chilli powder
- Salt to taste
- 1 tsp cumin seeds
- 2 tsp ginger garlic paste
- ¼ cup yoghurt
- 1 tbsp oil
- 1 tbsp dried fenugreek leaves
- Water (if required)

For pulao:

- 2.5 cups basmati rice (cooked)
- 1 cup vegetables (carrot, French beans, capsicum)
- 2 tsp cumin seeds
- 1 tbsp oil or ghee
- 2 bay leaves
- 2 cloves

- 2 dried red chillies
- 2 green chillies (chopped)
- ½ tsp red chilli powder
- 4 green cardamoms
- 2 black cardamoms
- 2 inch strips cinnamon sticks
- 1 onion (sliced)
- 1 tsp roasted cumin powder
- ¼ tsp garam masala powder
- Fresh coriander leaves (chopped)
- Salt to taste

Method:

For gattas:

1. Take a large mixing bowl.
2. Add gram flour, asafoetida, turmeric powder, red chilli powder, salt, cumin seeds, ginger-garlic paste, yoghurt, oil, dried fenugreek leaves and knead into a stiff dough.
3. Use 2 tbsp of water, if needed.
4. Divide the dough into 4–6 equal portions and shape each portion into 10-inch-long cylindrical rolls.
5. Boil enough water in a pan. Add rolls to the boiling water and boil for 10 to 15 minutes.
6. Remove from heat.
7. Take out the rolls from the water and keep the water aside for the curry base.
8. Cut each cylinder into 10–12 pieces, and keep aside.
9. Gattas are ready.

For pulao:

- Heat 1 tbsp oil in a deep non-stick pan. Add cumin seeds and let them splutter for a few seconds.
- Now add green cardamom pods, black cardamom, cloves, cinnamon sticks, red chillies, green chillies, bay leaf and sauté on medium heat for 30 seconds. Add onions and sauté until golden brown.
- Add vegetables and cook till soft.
- Add cooked gattas and sauté them for about 3–4 minutes.
- Add cooked rice, fried onions, chilli powder, turmeric powder, garam masala and salt, and mix well.
- Cook on medium heat for 3–4 minutes. Stir occasionally.
- Remove from heat.

Notes:

- Rice contains no gluten, hence can be consumed by the ones who are gluten-sensitive.
- Carrot sharpens your eyesight.
- Carrots also improve the appearance of skin, hair and nails.
- French beans are rich in iron, the nutrient found in haemoglobin that helps increase energy.
- French beans also help improve the immune system of the body as they are a rich source of vitamin C.
- Capsicum contains vitamins A and C, and beta-carotene that helps treat heart diseases, osteoarthritis, bronchial asthma and cataract.
- Capsicum increases metabolism due to capsaicin content.

Nutrition Table:

Calories (kcal)	Carbohydrates (g)	Protein (g)	Fat (g)
374	31	10	10

A Few Healthy Variations of Western Recipes

Peanut and Assorted Nut Butters

Ingredients:

- 100 gm peanuts

Method:

Roast peanuts (if raw) on a slow flame till the skins crack and place them in a grinder. Grind until it turns into butter.

Shredded Cheese

Ingredients:

- ½ cup soaked cashews
- 2 tbsp isabgul (psyllium husk)
- 4–5 garlic cloves
- 2 tbsp lemon juice
- ¼ cup water
- 1½ tsp rock salt
- A pinch of turmeric

Method:

Place all the ingredients in a grinder and blend until it forms a smooth paste. Transfer into a glass bowl, refrigerate for 6–8 hours. Cut into long shreds of cheese.

No-Bean Hummus

Ingredients:

- 2 cups zucchini
- ½ cup roasted white sesame seeds
- Lemon juice to taste
- 1 clove garlic (optional)
- 6–8 green olives
- 1 tsp paprika

Method:

Blend everything until smooth and serve.

Guidelines for Healthy Living

- Make sure you drink 3 litres of water daily. Use a glass or steel jar for drinking water. Note: Avoid adding lemon or any sour component in a copper vessel.

- Use cold pressed virgin coconut oil, unrefined rice bran, sesame, groundnut or mustard oil for Indian cooking. Extra virgin olive oil is to be added raw to salads.

- Have a salad or soup before your main course to feel partially full.

- There should be no more than 3–4 hours gap between each meal.

- Maintain a gap of 2.5 to 3 hours between dinner and bedtime; eating just before bedtime will cause acidity and heartburn.

- Eat mindfully. Chew your food well, eat slowly for a good 20 minutes, place your spoon or fork on the table after every bite, take deep breaths, and enjoy your meal. Make sure you stop once you've satiated yourself. The exhale should be a little longer than the inhale. Fast eating can trigger flatulence and bloating.

- Get at least 7–8 hours of sleep. Spend 10–15 minutes practising deep breathing before you hit the bed. Oxygen suppresses cortisol (stress hormone) and improves the quality of sleep.

- Avoid soya and its products (soya flour, soya bean, soya

granules, soya chunks, etc.), as it is known to cause hormonal imbalance.

- Keep all light-emitting gadgets away an hour before you sleep. Exposure to artificial light decreases melatonin, the sleep hormone.

- Stay active to keep your metabolism going! Be regular with your cardio and strengthening workouts.

- Avoid being sedentary for too long. Take a break every 45 minutes to an hour and walk around. 10,000 steps a day is a great way to improve metabolism. Move, stretch, walk, and take deep breaths whenever you can at frequent intervals.

- If you plan to eat out, drink a glass of vegetable juice beforehand. When choosing a meal at a restaurant, stick to the GPRS Mantra, i.e. Grilled/Poached/Roasted/Steamed or Stir-fried.

- Keep the portions in check. Slow eating will help with portion control. Serve yourself 1–2 tbsp lesser than usual.

- Besides your diet plan, eat fruits whenever you feel hungry. This works better than fruit juices. Avoid fruits after sunset as this interferes with sugar levels and digestion.

- The salt intake shouldn't exceed 1 tsp a day. Make use of herbs and spices to enhance flavour. Dried rosemary, oregano, dill, thyme, tamarind, lemon, cinnamon and nutmeg do a great job of adding flavour to the food and take care of our salt cravings!

- Try and minimize fatty foods and fried items.

- Avoid spicy and salty food like French fries, fried chips, spicy wafers, papads, pickles, etc.

- Avoid bakery products like biscuits, toast, pav, white bread, khari, etc. (to avoid excess trans fat, saturated fat, baking soda). These are not good for the liver and heart.

- Avoid processed food and refined sugar as it interferes with blood glucose level. Refined sugar triggers the release of inflammatory messengers called cytokines that aggravate pain. Avoid brown sugar and synthetic sweeteners as well; they are worse than sugar.

- Go for raw, unheated, unpasteurized honey or jaggery or dried stevia leaves instead.

- Keep your body alkaline (through lemon water, cucumbers, barley grass, green vegetables, aloe vera, etc.) to keep acidity at bay. It's always best to stay alkaline. Fat burns better in an alkaline medium.

- Cut down on tea and coffee. Apart from being acidic, tea and coffee tend to dehydrate our cells. Have a glass of water after every cup to rehydrate.

- Drink lemon water regularly. It's the most alkaline fruit! Avoid aerated drinks completely as they load your body with sugar and acid. Replace Coke with lemon water.

- Keep your bowels clean at all times. Constipation can lead to a build-up of toxins. Keep your motions smooth by consuming adequate fluids, water, good fats and coconut oil. 1 tbsp cold pressed castor oil at night with warm water can alleviate constipation. Avoid all synthetic laxatives.

- In case of sweet cravings, go for healthy sweet substitutes like dates or date rolls, 80 per cent dark chocolate, jaggery-based nut chikkis, dry fruit laddoos, ragi laddoos, etc. Keep a check on portions, 1 marble-sized or 1 inch square is best.

- Avoid plasticware. Avoid microwave or air fryer for cooking.

- Use steel/organic mud/glass vessels for cooking purposes.

- Use a cold press juicer for making vegetable juice.
- It is important to get rid of environmental toxins such as BPA that interfere with insulin receptors. Stop using plastic bottles. Switch to copper or glass or mud/clay pots to store water.
- Keep all light emitting gadgets away one hour before sleep, as light decreases melatonin, the sleep hormone.
- Indulge in deep breathing and meditation, either in the morning or at night.
- Expose yourself to sunlight as it is the best source of vitamin D.
- Inch loss is better than weight loss on the scale. Stay focused on fat loss (inch loss).

Conclusion

'Preserving our roots is like conserving the gene pool. If no one chronicles these age-old practices, all will be lost down the line.'

At some point, in the relentless quest for modernity, Indian habits stopped being cool. We've started believing that consuming only salads and soups is the way to a fit body, and having a car raises the standard of living. Moreover, popping a pill as a shortcut to reduce discomfort is like eating candy. This has resulted in an abandoning of traditional practices.

Pulses, legumes, rice grains, spinach, oils, ghee, millets are all looked down upon as being unnecessary for a calorie-conscious society. This has resulted in deficiencies of the body, increased discomfort and lifestyle-related disorders due to the lack of important minerals and vitamins. Diabetes, hypertension, thyroid issues and liver problems have begun to plague society. Popping of multivitamins, antacids, etc. has become so normal that people have forgotten to look for natural solutions inside the kitchens of their childhood.

In recent years, the same western diets have started incorporating ghee, virgin coconut oil, moringa, turmeric, ashwagandha, ginger and so many other Ayurvedic substances that have long since been an important part of Indian culture.

Turmeric latte has put the spotlight on a traditional Indian household drink, haldi doodh. Next in line is the humble drumstick. Moringa has become a new superfood, but Indians have been consuming cooked moringa and adding drumsticks in sambhar and gravies for ages. Unfortunately, we tend to think of our native foods as inferior until we receive validation to the contrary from abroad.

To be honest, cough syrups are no match for the traditional kadha lovingly prepared by our grandmothers.

Neem, tulsi, pepper and honey are ingredients that have always been consumed in India to build immunity and keep coughs and colds at bay. These native foods do more than just help us fight diseases; they build a nutritional bank that can take care of our entire bodies.

Our heritage needs to come back in a big way.

It has become the need of the hour for us to understand naturally available items that can be consumed throughout the year.

We have to get back to our roots in order to find health cures for diseases that plague our society.

We need to get back to the roots to prevent health issues.

We need to get back to the roots to let every cell in our body breathe to the fullest.

We need to get back to the roots for emotional stability!

We need to get back to the roots to rid ourselves of depression and anxiety!

We need to get back to the roots to raise the human consciousness!

We need to get back to the roots as it is a tool for well-being!

We need to get back to the roots as it is backed by science!

We need to get back to the roots as it is engineered with gentleness!

We need to get back to the roots for its incredibly rich heritage!